Ageless Beauty

An Insider's Guide to Advanced
Alternatives to Plastic Surgery

Ageless Beauty

An Insider's Guide to Advanced Alternatives to Plastic Surgery

Alexander J. Covey, M.D.

Mill City Press, Inc.
212 3rd Avenue North, Suite 290
Minneapolis, MN 55401
612.455.2294
www.millcitypublishing.com

ISBN - 978-1-934937-96-9
ISBN - 1-934937-96-7
LCCN - 2009929594

Cover Design by Jenni Wheeler
Typeset by James Arneson

Printed in the United States of America

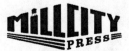

To my wife Lisa, my sons Michael and Jonathan, and my parents Dr. Alan and Sylvia Covey, all of whom have given me the pride and joy of my life. I also wish to thank my dedicated and wonderful staff and my loyal and extraordinary patients.

Table of Contents

Section Three
Summing It All Up

Appendices

Introduction

Helping to Turn Back the Clock

When I wrote my book "Forget the Knife: A Complete Guide to Cosmetic Rejuvenation Without Surgery" three years ago, I knew I was taking a chance that in its form as a complete guide it was going to be outdated almost immediately. And sure enough, the spring after "Forget the Knife" was published a new laser was introduced that promised skin resurfacing without downtime. Later that same laser was improved to include skin tightening, a new filler with promising results came out in the fall and was given FDA approval the next spring, and a new gentle light source was developed to help maintain the natural glow of younger looking skin. These were just a few of many advances.

Needless to say a plan for a new updated book was made. In reviewing "Forget the Knife" I realized that most of the nonsurgical treatments I introduced to you then are still leaders in the world of cosmetic treatments because they WORK! So what I decided to do is give you a refreshed, updated version of the first edition of "Forget the Knife" that includes the newest treatment options available.

Some of you may notice that I did not change a word in a few of the chapters. That's because the information, such as how to create and maintain a healthy lifestyle, is no different today than it was three years ago. But some of the chapters needed updating to include the newest effective treatments such as Thermage *which has been dramatically improved to give amazing results for your whole body, not just your face, and the revolutionary Fraxel re:pair Laser Treatment that was FDA approved for nonsurgical skin resurfacing and tightening just after the publication of "Forget The Knife."*

My hope is that this guide will help you in discovering the many ways you can look and feel your very best using the latest in proven, nonsurgical treatments for your face and body...so let's begin...

You know them when you see them, and you see them every day. They are the people who exude confidence and look younger than they are. They are the ones who look rested and refreshed even though they have the same kind of crazy schedules that we all do these days. Sometimes they are the strangers who smile at you across the display of grapefruit at the supermarket or help you at the retail store. Often, they are your acquaintances, co-workers, friends, and family members. And, they all have a secret.

They are all making use of new revolutionary advances that help "turn back the clock" to reduce signs of aging, skin damage, acne, rosacea, the ravages of the sun and smoking, and a wide range of other conditions in order to obtain a more youthful and polished appearance. When you know that you look your best, it reflects in your body language, presentation, and day-to-day life. While no health professional can ever truly make promises, these treatments can change the way you think about yourself and your life.

The scientific miracles available today are very different from the treatments, lotions, and potions of the past that made outrageous claims that they could never deliver. Instead, these products, procedures, and technologies offer proven success. They require little or no downtime, are often pain free, and are available at a reasonable cost with exceptional value. It is as close as you can get to Ponce de Leon's "Fountain of Youth" for anyone who has a desire to improve his or her appearance without going under the knife.

It should be said that there is nothing wrong with invasive surgical procedures. For some problems and for some people, these more drastic approaches are the right choice. Only your doctor can tell you if the results that you want can be accomplished without surgery. If, however, you are like most people, you want to explore all of the noninvasive alternatives before making a decision to try surgery.

By using some of the state-of-the-art nonsurgical procedures, products, and treatments outlined here, you may be able to achieve the results that you are seeking, hold off on radical surgical procedures, and get the satisfaction of knowing that you look your best and radiate confidence.

Looking great cannot be the responsibility of your doctor alone. You need to be an active participant in being the best that you can be. That means maintaining good general health, nutrition and dietary habits, and exercising regularly. That does not mean turning your life upside down, but it does suggest that, when you are considering these cosmetic procedures, it is also an appropriate time to take a broad look at your lifestyle and make any changes to behaviors that might put this new you at risk.

I have designed this book so that you can read it from cover to cover, which I encourage, since it can help you recognize your own areas of concern and get the full picture of the options that are available to solve them. It is also divided into sections that allow you to seek out specific treatments that can be matched with an individual subject that you may want to explore.

This book covers the topics that I am asked about most often, including lasers and other light source treatments, Botox, injectable fillers, nonsurgical face-lifts and body-lifts, mesotherapy and lipodissolve, acne and acne scarring, treatments for men, and information on home skin care so you can maintain your great looks.

It is also filled with information, suggestions, and stories of real people who have had success with the nonsurgical procedures that I discuss. Since the cosmetic procedure and product field changes almost daily, we encourage you to ask your doctor about anything that is so new that it might not be included here. Never be afraid to ask what's new.

Simply put, my objective is to:

- Make you an educated person who uses the best technology and your skin's power of renewal to maintain a healthy, youthful appearance throughout your life
- Teach you about the behaviors that put your face and body at risk and how to avoid them
- Choose procedures, treatments, and products that fit your particular needs
- Encourage you to take good care of yourself in all aspects including nutrition and exercise, so that you can get the greatest value from state-of-the-art rejuvenation technology
- Build an understanding of how you can take full advantage of the wide variety of noninvasive breakthroughs in anti-aging treatments that have emerged in recent years.

I have laid out the information that you will need to know about the exciting new techniques and solutions that can help you create a powerful program for optimizing your appearance and well-being and that can make you one of those self-assured people who love the way they look and always look their very best.

Taking Care of Yourself

CHAPTER 1

Healthy Lifestyle:

The Right Fuel for a Beautiful Machine

With all of the wonderful new noninvasive treatments and procedures available today and in the future, one thing remains true: your lifestyle (nutrition and exercise) is a key factor in maintaining your skin and keeping your youthful appearance.

Unhealthy habits, notably excessive tanning, too much alcohol and smoking, poor eating, and a lack of physical activity can have a negative impact on how you feel and how you look. You don't need to run marathons or triathlons and stick to a diet of sprouts and nuts. Rather, it's about providing the fuel that keeps all of your systems operating at peak efficiency.

Think of it this way: when you make the decision to purchase a fabulous new car, you read the manual about the right gas, oil, and other fuels and additives, and about how to operate the vehicle for both long life and optimal performance. That is what your warranty is based upon. When you handle scratches, dents, and other small problems on a timely basis, you keep them from becoming big problems.

People don't come with warranties, but the same concept

applies. For long life and optimal performance, there are certain rules. If you follow them, the results are usually excellent for your entire body. The added benefit is that your skin loves the same things as the rest of your body systems. Plenty of water, the improved circulation that exercise provides, and great eating habits pay off in youthful, healthy looking skin.

The dents and dings on a car are comparable to those hated skin problems that make you look older and more tired than you really are. For them, your doctor is the best resource. With the alternatives, from VolumaLifts to Thermage and Botox injections, a full range of laser treatments, and other products and procedures, almost every problem has a solution designed to keep you young and vibrant looking.

Exercise for a Healthier, Better-Looking You

You can hardly open a newspaper, read a magazine, or watch television without reading something about the importance of a weekly exercise routine. Some researchers actually say that nutrition and exercise can sometimes be the equivalent of medical treatments because of their impact on many physical, emotional, and mental conditions, including heart disease, strokes, and some cancers. When it comes to aging, exercise can also reverse some of the effects and combat diseases such as diabetes, osteoporosis, and arthritis.

In regards to the skin, exercise improves muscle tone, making the skin look smoother by stimulating the flow of blood and providing nutrients. You may have actually seen it when you looked in the mirror after a healthy workout and saw the glow that came from inside. If you are honest with yourself, you have also seen a younger, healthier reflection.

And, since there is such a close mind-body relationship, you tend to feel the results of exercise in a reduced stress level and a general feeling of well-being. You can attribute that to the endorphins that your body produces. (Chocolate also has some of the same effect, but a body can only take so much of a good thing.)

There are three kinds of exercise and, if possible, it is best to fit each of them into your routine:

- Aerobic exercise raises your pulse rate and increases the flow of oxygen throughout your body. You can get it from a brisk thirty-minute walk or some structured exercise programs.
- Strength or resistance exercise keeps the muscles in tone and increases breathing capabilities. Whether you work out with machines, free weights, or a couple of large soup cans, ten minutes a day or more can make a real difference in how you look and feel.
- Flexibility training increases your flexibility through stretches that loosen the muscles and keep body movements fluid.

There are cautions that you should take with starting an exercise program. After years of inactivity, it takes time to condition the body to a new routine. It is always recommended to talk to your physician and work with an exercise specialist or trainer—even if only to get a good start.

Only you can be responsible for maintaining the exercise program once you have begun. To keep things interesting, vary your activities. There are many alternatives for each of the three exercise types. This is one case where variety is the spice of life.

Feeding the Body Means Feeding the Skin

It seems difficult to comprehend, but everything you put into your body shows up in your skin. That is why people with poor diets often have pasty, mottled, or otherwise unattractive skin.

Healthy skin tone and diet are connected. Just as the other body systems rely on the nutrients from the foods you eat, so does the skin. More importantly, unlike all of those internal systems, this one helps determine how other people perceive you. It's a fact that people who eat properly often find that their skin appearance improves and that the change to a healthier diet can help to reverse the signs of aging.

Fruits and vegetables lead the way to healthy, vibrant skin. They are readily available sources of vitamins, minerals, and phytochemicals (phyto means plant in Greek) that help to enhance cell repair and renewal. This action at the cellular level is important because these naturally occurring chemicals help to keep a balance and protect the body—especially the skin—from breaking down at the cellular level. The science is quite complex but all evidence points to this as being one of the factors in aging.

The Best Alternatives

A healthy diet doesn't need to be boring. Unless you are completely committed to a junk food diet, you are sure to find a range of healthy foods that provide the nutrients that have the most positive impact on your skin.

The list of foods that do the most for you has been recited many times and I won't detail it here. It does bear repeating, however, that a few are standouts. Whole grains; green, leafy vegetables; broccoli; asparagus; salmon and other fish high in Omega-3 fatty acids; chicken; fruits—especially dark berries, cantaloupes, citrus, and tropical fruits like mangoes; and some dairy products should be the basis of your regular diet. However, watch your portions, since too much of a good thing is not a good thing.

Many of the foods that people love, including beef, are not on this list. It doesn't mean that you need to give them up entirely, but you are encouraged to make good choices and have the beef, sweets, and desserts as the exception rather than the rule for your everyday regimen.

The most important nutrients for your skin are vitamins A, B, C, and E; copper; selenium; zinc; coenzyme Q10—important as an anti-aging oxidant; and alpha lipoic acid, which stimulates collagen repair. All of these can be found in supplements but supplements should be used only when you can't get the minimum daily requirement in your diet. That said, a multivitamin and mineral supplement taken each day is an easy way to ensure that you get the right amount of everything.

For prepared foods, read the labels and be an educated consumer. For example, almost every mention of oil or syrup in a list of ingredients translates to fat or sugar. Look out for trans fats and avoid them.

Remember that the scientific thinking is changing so rapidly about good eating alternatives and minimum daily requirements that it is always good to ask your doctor about what is best for you.

The Fountain of Youth

The next time you walk past a drinking fountain or miss the opportunity to have a refreshing drink of water, you are missing out on a dip into the fountain of youth. Water helps skin maintain its moisture content and helps to minimize the look of fine lines and wrinkles. The combination of water plus the treatments, procedures, and products that your doctor offers for skin rejuvenation are a great one-two punch for staying younger looking and healthy.

Don't wait to be thirsty to drink water. Your body generally doesn't signal that you are dehydrated until you are down about five percent from what your water balance should be.

Summing It Up

Exercise, diet, and adequate hydration are important elements in maintaining good skin tone and good health. When you combine them with the easy, noninvasive alternatives that your doctor can offer you, there is no reason to look any other way than great.

CHAPTER 2

Beautiful Skin:
A Realistic Goal

How would you describe the most beautiful skin that you have ever seen? For most people, the word that comes to mind is "flawless." While it is usually an overstatement since almost everyone's skin has imperfections, the perception is what counts. If you could do what it takes so others have that perception of you, wouldn't you do it? And, if you could do it in seven steps over a thirty day period with extraordinary results, wouldn't that be even more tempting?

This is no idle daydream. It is a realistic goal that can be achieved by combining your desire and commitment with the skills and knowledge of a board certified specialist in cosmetic procedures. It can't be done with the array of lotions and potions on the market today, but you probably know that already. Most people try these first and few are ever satisfied with the results. Product promises generally don't produce the beautiful skin that you are seeking—even when combined with all the wishful thinking in the world.

You are not alone in your quest. Men and women both express their disappointment with treatments that they have tried or the way that their skin has aged and changed.

"I always took good care of my skin. I watch my diet and exercise, but my skin never looks as good as I feel inside. I can't believe I still have to deal with pimples at my age."

Kathy F., age 32, Nurse

"I play a lot of golf. Over the years, I've had a great deal of skin exposure and now my skin is getting rougher and I'm noticing more wrinkles than ever before."

Stacey M., age 44, Teacher

"I always get flushed and have a very red face. I'm also beginning to get these thick red veins on my nose and lots of brown spots on my face and hands."

Richard T., age 56, Lawyer

In recent years, science and technology have come a long way toward determining the causes for these problems and many other skin concerns. Now there are solutions that can make a real difference in how you feel about yourself and how others see you.

Seven Steps to Beautiful Skin

There are seven simple things that you can do with little or no expense to improve your skin.

1. Wear Sunscreen Every Day

The sun shines every day, whether you see it peeking from behind a cloud or beating down in ninety-degree heat. You are out in it even when you dart out from your car to the store or sit behind the steering wheel or in the passenger seat of a car. You can't escape it entirely, and—as you have heard and read in all of the media—sun damage is the enemy of your skin. No matter how good it makes you feel, sun exposure is not your friend.

The effects of sun exposure are cumulative. Your skin is like the elephant that never forgets, and the result can be a dull, leathery appearance; wrinkles and lines; brown spots; and the highly visible blood vessels on your skin. If you doubt this, compare the skin on your inner forearm with that of the skin on the back of your hand or other exposed area of your skin.

The scientific experts say, and I agree, that you should use sunscreen every day. Apply it often, too. Much of the current research has shown that the frequency with which you apply sunscreen is as important as a higher SPF level.

Sunscreens work their best if you apply them indoors about thirty minutes before you go outside, allowing them to dry first. But don't forget to reapply them if you are going to spend much time outdoors; their efficiency does decrease over time.

I am often asked if it is really necessary to throw away sunscreen after one year, as the manufacturers recommend, or if it is simply a way to sell more products. The truth is that most sunscreens are good for two years or so, although they may be a bit less potent. The real reason to discard them after a year is that the opening and closing of the container, its proximity to the beach and other outdoor venues, and other situations can allow them to become contaminated. If you are using the one or two ounces that the manufacturers recommend for the initial application each day, there will be very little to discard anyway.

For women, many facial foundations contain a minimum of SPF 15 sunscreen as one of their features. This is not enough for outside activities on very sunny days, but it is a start. This is a good way to kill two birds with one stone, as the old saying goes.

If you have sun damage already, talk to your doctor about reversing its effects. And remember that if you revert to your old habits after undertaking treatment for the damage, the blemishes may return. It is a matter of changing your habits.

2. Stop Smoking NOW and Cut Down on Drinking Alcohol

Like sun damage, smoking has a cumulative effect on your skin. Drinking alcohol does as well. If you are a smoker who is unhappy with the fine lines, wrinkles, and condition of your skin, you already know the culprit. Smoking is the one thing that virtually every medical professional, journal, and expert say is bad for your health. There is a reason why: tobacco is the leading cause of lung cancer—one of the most lethal cancers in our world today—and one that you may be able to prevent to some extent. It is not easy to quit, but the payoff is well worth it.

Drinking, too, affects your skin and its appearance. Alcohol tends to expand your blood vessels, causing red spots on your skin. If you know a heavy drinker, you have probably seen this as they have aged. Some people say that they can recognize a drinker by these red spots, which can appear extensive. While there are multiple reasons for red spots, alcohol consumption is one of the most common. Unlike smoking, merely cutting down on drinking does help, even if you do not give it up entirely.

As with sun damage, there are procedures and treatments that can improve your appearance and repair some of the damage caused by smoking and drinking. First, however, it is important to modify your habits so that your improved appearance after working with your doctor will be long lasting. Going back to bad habits means giving up the ground that you have won by dealing with your skin problems.

3. Drink Plenty of Water

You have probably read or heard that most of your body is fluid. Drinking as much water as possible through the course of every day helps to keep the balance that your system requires. It helps to keep your skin clear and all of the subsystems operating at peak efficiency.

Those folks who you see toting around sipping cups or bottles of water already know this, and many of them have the healthy hydrated look to their skin that you admire. Take a cue from them by drinking six to ten cups of water every day.

Remember, too, that caffeinated beverages do not count toward your water intake. Caffeine is a drug that makes your body get rid of water and can contribute to dehydration.

4. Exercise for Good Health and Healthy Skin

There is not necessarily the need to "feel the burn," although it is a sign of a good workout. Our bodies were not designed to be constantly sedentary. They were designed for movement and activity, and exercise is one way to bring it into our lives.

Exercise raises our spirits by releasing endorphins (so does eating a bit of dark chocolate, but that is definitely a reward rather than a replacement) and bringing much-needed oxygen into our systems. Exercise also increases blood circulation to the skin, along with the added oxygen and nutrients, making us look better.

This is not a one time deal. Create an exercise plan that you can live with and that offers strength training, aerobic activity, and flexibility aspects. Make it fun, if you can, so you don't get tired of the routine. Increase your exercise activity as it becomes too easy, while keeping it within guidelines that you and your doctor or trainer recommends. Overexertion, especially as we age, can sour us on exercise entirely.

Remember that dancing is a great way to exercise. It can give you a good workout if you commit to it and, rumor has it, a good fox trot, salsa, or tap dance can keep you smiling while you stretch those muscles.

Don't build your exercise plan around activities that you hate or you will always find an excuse to avoid it. There is a great deal of variety out there. It may take a little research to find out what works for you, but it is worth the effort. Create small rewards (not food or alcohol) to mark exercise milestones.

5. Reduce Stress

This is the toughest challenge among my seven steps. Stress is very bad for your body and skin. It can indirectly affect your hormonal system, leading to skin problems like breakouts, acne, wrinkles, and frown lines.

Some stressful things we cannot avoid, but we can often cushion ourselves from the worst of it. First, do an honest evaluation of the things and situations that cause stress in your life. Second, write it all down to make it real, and be both frank and detailed. Put the list away for a day or two and return to it when you have time to really evaluate the items.

The probability is that you will find some of them are out of your control. If you are dealing with illness, either yours or that of someone close to you, that is a good example. At the same time, look at how many of the items are either caused or aggravated by you.

We often increase our stress level by taking on more than we can realistically achieve, aiming only at the top when getting there by consistent baby steps is a better choice, or being driven by work, religious, or community commitments. Take a deep breath and learn to make time for yourself.

Whether it is a soak in a bubble bath, a walk through a lovely place, quiet meditation, a good book, or something that only you know minimizes stress, plan it into your day—every day. Behavioral experts even say that petting a dog or cat reduces stress for many people. If you are not sure what activities are stress reducers for you personally, make a list of all the things that you enjoy. If you are at a loss, think of *The Sound of Music* hit, "My Favorite Things," and use it as a start. After all, who doesn't like raindrops on roses?

6. Get Enough Sleep

This is like recharging your batteries and it can provide an instant lift. It takes six to eight hours a night to obtain and maintain a fresh and healthy look. It will also reduce your puffy eyes and tired look, as well as discouraging that frequent and unattractive yawning.

Here are some tips for getting that wonderful night's rest:

- Don't eat late at night. It can keep you awake.
- Do your exercising earlier in the day. While it seems as though intensive activity should make you tired enough to fall asleep more quickly, most people find it doesn't work that way.
- No caffeine after dinner; it is a stimulant.
- Establish a routine bedtime and stick with it when you can.
- Create at least half an hour of quiet time before getting into bed. Reading or listening to music will relax you. Some people like to do yoga during this pre-bedtime period.
- If you have problems with insomnia, talk to your medical doctor about holistic remedies and prescription products that are not habit forming.

7. Maintain a Good Skin Care Regimen

If you neglect your skin, it will look tired and worn, and any imperfections will become more obvious. Keeping it clean is a great defense. Remove dirt, oil, makeup, and dead skin cells with products that are designed for those purposes. Moisturize often. It doesn't replace the noninvasive treatments and procedures in this book, but it will help you to maintain that youthful, rejuvenated appearance.

Routine care can make the difference between skin that looks dull and clogged, and a fresh hydrated look. It also helps to minimize pimples and other imperfections—those little thieves of your self-confidence. This is something that you can do for yourself. Your doctor can make appropriate recommendations for your particular skin type or problem areas.

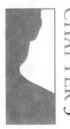

CHAPTER 3

Just for Men:
Literally Everything

You have probably noticed that this is not a long chapter. It really doesn't need to be since *everything* in this book is for you if you are a man, or for every male spouse, parent, friend, acquaintance, or business associate who wants to look younger and healthier or who needs to solve a skin problem.

There was a time when the procedures described in this book, along with many others classified as "cosmetic," were seen only as being for women. Those days are gone. Every year for which statistical analysis is done clearly shows that more and more men are being proactive in addressing unwanted hair, skin problems, and rejuvenation with the same range of extraordinary alternatives that women have always recognized. In fact, men represent the greatest growth of any group.

There are good reasons for this. This is one place where there is none of the men-versus-women controversy. Men are subject to the same unwanted hair, acne and acne scarring, age spots, rosacea, and the effects of aging and bad habits that affect women. In many cases, because men have been less attentive to their skin as they age, they have far worse cases of sun damage and other problems.

Men have typically had the advantage of the world seeing the rugged outdoorsman with a lined face and sun-weathered skin or the fellow with crow's feet from smiling into the sun at the helm of his boat as romantic characters. But many men are finding that the results of aging—including lines, deep wrinkles, and loss of collagen—simply make them look old and tired.

Many research studies have found that a young looking man is more apt to be seen as dynamic and progressive in the business world and that both women and men respond more positively to a man that obviously takes care of his appearance.

While every procedure mentioned in this book may meet your specific needs, a consultation with a respected doctor who specializes in this field will design a plan for regaining that rejuvenated image and address your specific skin problems that cause discomfort or embarrassment.

Among the most popular procedures and treatments to discuss with your doctor are

- Contouring your face and body with Smartlipo
- Help for active acne and acne scarring including resurfacing, laser and light treatments, and dermal fillers
- Acne and rosacea care that can include multiple treatments to keep the problem under control
- Fine lines and all kinds of wrinkles that can be treated with Botox, dermal fillers including Restylane, Juvederm, Radiesse, Evolence and VolumaLift, Thermage and Fraxel lasers for a full-face nonsurgical lift
- Fat removal with mesotherapy and lipodissolve (including those love handles and multiple chins) that

won't go away even with a regular exercise and diet regime

- Removal of dark spots, freckles, and other skin imperfections
- Laser hair removal for unwanted hair
- A range of solutions for maintaining a healthy, attractive appearance.

If you believe you could look better but have no desire for a surgical solution that can cause downtime, discomfort, and permanent results that you may not like but which cannot easily be reversed, these solutions are for you. (Did you know that about fifty percent of most plastic surgeons' business is corrective surgery to repair something for the dissatisfied patient of another doctor?)

All of the treatments, procedures, and solutions described in this book require little or no downtime. You will see that none of these are addressed specifically to women because they are not simply the problems of women. Everyone today is conscious of the importance of his or her appearance and the perception of others.

As with women, it is also critical that you work with a doctor who has treated men and can show you the results. Together you can develop a program that will result in the healthy, rejuvenated appearance that you want and need to stay happy in this highly competitive world.

Section Two

Cosmetic Treatments
That Can Help You

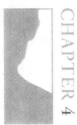

CHAPTER 4

Botox:

The Modern Miracle

If Coca-Cola is the world's most recognized brand name, Botox is quickly gaining ground. In a very short time it has become part of our day-to-day vocabulary, even though it is a brand name for a highly specialized product that you can't buy at any store.

Why? The answer is easy. Botox has become a household name because it is a product that works. People all over the world have welcomed a way to make facial wrinkles disappear, to wipe away frown lines, and to erase the years without surgery.

At the same time, research has shown that this drug is an excellent treatment for excessive armpit sweating and migraine headaches. Its success has been documented, and researchers are always on the lookout for new ways to use it.

It is no wonder that about 4.6 million people are treated with Botox every year, making it one of the most frequently requested procedures in the world and the most commonly performed minimally invasive procedure.

Today it is a popular game to look at photos and film of famous people, including Hollywood stars, and ask the question: Are they using Botox? While few people admit to it, the probability is that if you see a subtle yet impressive difference in their facial appearance, they are probably having Botox treatments. If they look rested and relaxed without crow's-feet, forehead furrows, and worry lines, they probably are having Botox injections. It they look younger and more refreshed, even with hectic schedules and time commitments, they are probably having Botox. They may never tell and when you make the decision to try Botox, you won't have to tell anyone either.

To determine whether you are ready to start a Botox regimen, see if you fit the following scenario.

You arrive at work feeling as though you had a great night's sleep. You are ready to attack the day and you feel refreshed and energetic. It is a good hair day, your clothes look terrific, and you are wearing fabulous new shoes.

The bubble bursts, however, when you stop to say hi to the receptionist and she asks, "Are you feeling okay? You really look tired." Now, you are really worried. What happened between home and work? Is there something you missed?

You rush into the restroom and look in the mirror. You are a lot more critical this time. You do look tired. Your forehead and frown lines and the crow's-feet around your eyes are obvious. You feel good but your face doesn't reflect it; what a downer. You know this revelation will affect how you feel about yourself for the rest of the day and for many days to follow.

Think about it. When you admit it to yourself, you can't remember the last time you looked in the mirror and felt that you looked your best. You feel youthful and vibrant and lead a lifestyle that belies your age, but you are beginning to wonder what that face is telling others.

There have been many studies done over the years that showed that in a business or social environment, people respond more positively to those who look as though they feel good about themselves. Botox just may be the right tool for you to help build confidence and give you a competitive edge.

How Botox Works

Every expression and every emotion uses many tiny muscles in your face at the same time. This expressiveness makes us who we are, but years or decades of repeating these muscular contractions leave their mark in the form of wrinkles and furrows around your eyes, forehead, and other parts of your face. Botox works by relaxing these muscles and giving the appearance of softening lines and wrinkles. The value is in both the way these dynamic wrinkles are reduced and in the way that Botox treatment limits your ability to portray an angry, sad, or otherwise negative emotion. You look more relaxed, yet retain your ability to be expressive in the best ways possible.

A Brief History of Botox

Botox is not a new product. For about forty years, it has been used as a treatment for neurological problems. It provides relief for patients with diseases like cerebral palsy. It is used to treat crossed eyes, involuntary winking, and other illnesses that are caused by muscle spasms and similar conditions—not terribly glamorous, but highly effective. It wasn't until the late 1980s that the medical community saw the opportunity to use Botox for cosmetic procedures.

It was Dr. Jean Carruthers, a Canadian ophthalmologist, who saw the possibilities. While treating patients with eye conditions such as misaligned eyes, she found that the injections of Botox that she was giving also caused the lines around the eyes to vanish. Patients looked more relaxed and less angry.

Recognizing its unique potential, Dr. Carruthers, along with her husband, Dr. Alastair Carruthers, a dermatologist, decided to try it on his dermatology patients with amazing results. The word spread, papers were presented at conferences, and the manufacturer of Botox sought and received FDA approval for this new use. (Drugs must be approved by the FDA for new uses even though they have been approved before, and that was the case with Botox.)

Only Botox is Botox

Botox is a biological toxin (botulinum toxin type A) transformed into a therapeutic agent. It is the exclusive brand name of a single source, Allergan, which assures its quality. Only Botox *is* Botox.

Since the 1960s, genuine Botox has been used for a range of neurological disorders with excellent outcomes. But one result of ongoing research was the finding that when injected into the areas where facial lines form, Botox could help to turn back the clock. It has been used for cosmetic procedures for more than twenty years and is one of the fastest-growing solutions for anti-aging and rejuvenation.

Its uses are varied, and include correction of brow furrows and forehead lines, the appearance of a nonsurgical brow lift, smoothing of crow's-feet around the eyes, lip wrinkles and neck bands, and more. Botox is also used to reduce excessive armpit and hand sweating (believe it or not) and to treat migraine headaches.

Botox relaxes the underlying muscles to give a smooth, unwrinkled appearance so you have little more to do than accept the compliments on how rested and youthful you look.

The Procedure

Botox treatments take only a few minutes. A very small amount of the product is injected into the areas of concern using a very tiny needle. Because the needle is so fine and the amount of Botox so small, there is minimal discomfort involved.

No sedation or local anesthesia is necessary and you can resume your normal schedule immediately. If there is any bruising at the injection site, a touch of makeup should solve the problem.

Safety of Botox

In the hands of a seasoned medical professional, Botox is very safe to use. Over the years, there have been horror stories and one in particular has made the rounds for years.

In Florida, an unlicensed chiropractor used a "bootleg" version of Botox that was illegally imported from Mexico and never intended for use by humans. It was approximately one hundred times as powerful as cosmetic Botox, and it caused a serious disease.

There have been other cases where a diluted Botox product gave results that were not acceptable or long lasting. A reputable physician would never water down the product; but, if you have had Botox treatments that only lasted for a few weeks, diluted Botox could be the culprit. Don't look for Botox bargains or you may be disappointed.

In the millions of injections of Botox given year after year, the only reported side effects have been transient and minor. As with any medical procedure, it is recommended that you tell your doctor if you are taking any medications, and avoid taking things like vitamin E and aspirin (which can cause unnecessary bruising) for about a week before Botox treatments. It is not so much a safety issue as a tip that will make you look great even faster.

Questions, Questions, Questions

It is very logical for people to have concerns about a product that has received so much publicity and is so popular. Some questions are so frequently asked that we have answered them here. I encourage you to discuss them with your doctor and make sure that they are answered to your satisfaction before you undertake Botox treatments or any of the other procedures covered in this book.

1. How long will it last?

Every person is different, but Botox for facial wrinkles generally lasts three to six months. After a while, the interval for injections often becomes longer. When you feel that you need a treatment, you set up an appointment with your doctor for a very short session (usually five or ten minutes for the injections).

2. Is it possible to look worse if you stop Botox treatments?

You will not look worse if you stop Botox treatments. However, if you have had them for a long time, you may actually have forgotten how you looked before the lines and wrinkles vanished. There is no record of any patients having a "rebound" effect after stopping Botox. On the other hand, some patients even report long-lasting softening of their lines months after stopping their Botox.

3. Since Botox is a potent poison, why would I want to put it into my body?

It is true that Botox is a very potent medication that can do damage in the hands of an unqualified person. It can be inadvertently injected into the wrong place in the wrong amount. In the hands of an experienced physician who has had a good deal of experience with Botox, it should be injected properly and it is unlikely to cause any side effects.

Think of this as a comparison: Many heart medications are poisonous if they are improperly prescribed or if they are ingested in the wrong dosage. In the hands of a specialist, however, they can be life sustaining. Again, it is an issue of dosage and how it is used.

One way to avoid any problems is to look for the right doctor, ask the questions that you need answered to put your mind at ease, and be comfortable with that specialist's credentials. You can get a quick course on how to do this in Chapter 16.

4. Doesn't Botox make you look plastic or unnatural?

Anything taken to an unhealthy extreme is a problem. Botox is no exception. I am sure you have seen people, including movie stars, who have a frozen look without expression. This can be caused by too much Botox in too many places. But, how do you know when an amount is too much?

That is for the pros. If it is used tastefully, Botox will give you a relaxed look. The key is to know how far to go without temporarily over-weakening any of the essential muscles required for proper facial expression.

Again, this is where the judgment of your physician comes into play. You need to rely on the doctor's expertise, so select a practitioner who can assure you of natural-looking results.

5. If Botox treatments are so easy, why can't anyone do it?

While a terrific doctor can make Botox treatments look effortless, it takes considerable experience and knowledge of facial anatomy to evaluate where and how much Botox should be used. This is highly personalized for each patient.

Think of it this way: You have only one face. It precedes you before you say a word and it looks back at you from the mirror. Would you be willing to put your one-and-only face in the hands of someone other than the best?

6. Isn't Botox addictive?

For a drug to be addictive, it must pass appreciably into the blood stream or into the brain, having a systemic effect. Botox is a drug that has local effects and does not affect your body as a whole. Beyond the area where it is injected, it does not affect the nervous system.

The only addiction that is a risk is to the results—an improved, relaxed appearance that you will never want to give up.

7. Can Botox cause permanent eyelid droop?

The condition that you are asking about is called ptosis, or eyelid droop. It is a rarely seen complication and is generally avoidable with the proper technique and expertise.

Remember, all of Botox's effects are temporary and if in the unlikely case this were to occur, it would not be permanent. In fact, it usually resolves within a week or two. Additionally, it can be easily treated with special eye drops that reverse the problem. Permanent eyelid droop is not a concern.

8. Shouldn't I be satisfied with how I look as I age?

Never feel guilty when contemplating a cosmetic procedure like Botox. It doesn't actually change your appearance. You still look like yourself. Instead, it returns your looks to the way they used to be before all the stress and years added lines to your face. There is no age limit for wanting to look your best.

The Next Step

Look in the mirror once more. If you don't like what you see, set up an appointment for a consultation about Botox. This gives you an opportunity to hear the facts, get expert advice, and make an educated decision about whether Botox can improve your appearance and your confidence.

CHAPTER 5

Filling in the Blanks:
Dermal Fillers

How often have you read a line in a book that described the character by saying that his or her face fell? If you think back, it probably did not refer to the hero or heroine in good circumstances. Falls are great when they refer to waterfalls, an exquisite autumn, or falling in love. The rest of the time, you need to ask yourself how you feel about falling—especially when it refers to your face.

When you consider all of the effects that aging has on your skin, one of the most common—and most annoying—is the presence of deep lines, folds, furrows, and a loss of volume that seems to reflect every emotion or stress-inducing event that ever occurred in your life. While some people consider these features to be battle scars, and say that you haven't lived a meaningful life if you don't have furrows and wrinkles to show for it, many others have come to realize that you can embrace the meaning of life without wearing it on your face.

The fallen face and the deep lines and furrows are often the result of a loss of volume in the dermis and subcutaneous layers of the skin—two skin layers that lie below the surface layer. As we age; engage in unhealthy behaviors like smoking, tanning, and excessive drinking; and deal with everyday stress, the collagen and elastin that keep things looking tight and youthful deteriorate. In order to get that look back, something needs to replace the lost tissue and pump up the volume.

The medical community and scientists have been dealing with the question of how this should be done for more than a century. In the 1800s, researchers made the discovery that a patient's own body fat could be obtained and relocated to other parts of the body, including the face. Then paraffin was tried, but after twenty years or so, it was abandoned. Next followed silicone fillers, some of which are still in use today in a highly improved form. In the 1970s, California-based researchers first worked with bovine (cow) collagen as a filler material and, in 1981, this product (marketed as Zyderm) was granted FDA approval. It and two other forms of bovine collagen trademarked as Zyderm II and Zyplast were also approved. All are still in use, but many new products available today are growing in importance.

While there are many dermal filler options and new alternatives that are being added as soon as they receive government approval in the United States, this chapter deals with some of the more popular ones that provide excellent proven results. All are temporary fillers that offer the advantage of wearing away rather than having to sometimes be reversed by a second surgery if something is not up to your expectations.

As mentioned before, bovine (cow) collagen was among the first fillers used. It had drawbacks, however, including potential for an allergic reaction in about three percent of the population, making it necessary to perform a skin test twenty-eight days before treatment. It also had a very fast breakdown in the body, which made it a poor value for most people. While it has been improved and is still actively prescribed, there is now a wider range of solutions available including some with extraordinary results, but only your doctor can tell you which is right for you.

Is it any wonder then that the last decade has seen an exceptional amount of research in dermal fillers with excellent results that offer you and your doctor this range of choices for creating volume where you need it to fill lines and furrows? There have been so many developments, with new ones being announced on a regular basis, that it would be impossible to keep a book chapter completely up to date. The alternatives that are described here are among the most effective at the time of publication. They, too, are being researched for the longest-lasting and most successful results. Consult with your specialist to find out about the latest and greatest dermal fillers.

Determining Your Need for Dermal Fillers

You can determine if you are a good candidate for dermal fillers if you have any of the following facial problems:

- *Facial folds and lines that often stretch from the nose to the mouth.* We call them smile lines when we are young, but as we get older and the volume of collagen is depleted, they age us and make us look glum, tired, or sad.
- *Horizontal lines on the forehead that make a person look worried or concerned, even when he or she is not.*
- *Vertical lines that are just above the lip line (often extending into the lip line) and below the lower lip line.* These are the places where smokers and people who have tanned for

years often see problems. It is also the area that, if you are a lipstick wearer, the line becomes irregular and can make lipstick appear to bleed or look sloppy, even if the application is perfect to start with. Even without lipstick, these lines affect expression and make us look older.

- *Turndown at the corners of the mouth that often makes a person look angry or sullen, and they never seem to go away no matter how happy he or she is.*
- *A gaunt appearance that ages the face and makes a person look less vibrant and healthy.*
- *Under-eye darkness or bagginess that is visible because of the translucent appearance of the skin and a loss of collagen volume.*
- *Some scarring.* This is not the best solution for all scarring and your doctor may have other recommendations that will be more effective for you individually.

Some Current Fillers

The following are a few of the most popular fillers used today:

Restylane, Juvederm, and Perlane

Restylane has the highest profile of all dermal fillers. (Juvederm and Perlane are other hyaluronic acid dermal fillers.) These cosmetic dermal fillers are made of nonanimal stabilized hyaluronic acid. Hyaluronic acid exists in its natural form in the human body and is responsible for retaining water and elasticity in the skin. As we age, our own hyaluronic acid decreases; to remain younger looking, we must replace it.

Here's an interesting fast fact: as with many of the current procedures using state-of-the-art materials, synthetic hyaluronic acids, such as Restylane, were originally developed for use by orthopedic surgeons to improve joint function. Its uses today go far beyond that, and hyaluronic acid fillers have been used extensively for cosmetic treatments throughout the world.

One of Restylane's and other hyaluronic acid fillers' benefits is that as natural, animal-free, crystal clear gels that are biodegradable, there is no need for allergy testing and the great majority of people find that these are excellent solutions for filling lines and furrows or plumping lips that have lost their luxurious fullness.

The areas that generally respond best to treatment include the fine lines on the upper and lower lips, deeper wrinkles, and folds such as those in the nasolabial areas and the corners of the mouth. Acne scarring can be minimized with dermal fillers, and Perlane is often a perfect choice for lips, replacing the need for implants.

Treatments are completely nonsurgical, with the doctor injecting a tiny amount of filler with a very fine needle into each area. Results are immediate and get even better over time. There is no downtime at all and the effects are relatively long lasting. When there is a need for a touch-up, it can be done easily by your doctor in a few minutes. Unlike permanent implants or surgical solutions, you can always reverse the effect as the filler dissolves over time. However, with more than two million treatments since Restylane's introduction in 1996, the desire to reverse the effect is an extremely rare occurrence. It is far more likely that after experiencing the great results, you will decide to add more areas of treatment with these amazing products.

Radiesse

Radiesse is one of the newest nonsurgical facial contouring fillers available today. Many people find that this filler, made from very tiny smooth calcium hydroxylapatite (CaHa) lasts longer than other products—sometimes as long as two years with occasional touch-ups.

CaHa is a biomaterial that has been used for more than twenty years in orthopedics, neurosurgery, and ophthalmology and is the primary mineral constituent of bone and teeth. For Radiesse, this biomaterial is suspended in a common water-based carrier in clear gel form.

As with Restylane and other hyaluronic acid fillers, the visible improvement is immediate. And, like these well-established products, there is no need for pretesting with Radiesse. There is no downtime.

CosmoDerm and CosmoPlast

The manufacturers of these dermal fillers say that to see if collagen replacement therapy is right for you, simply perform a basic stretch test. Pull your skin tight on either side of the wrinkle that you want to evaluate for treatment. If the line or wrinkle goes away when the skin is stretched, then full correction can be achieved with their use. The line will remain but filling will get rid of the wrinkle and minimize the appearance by smoothing the skin.

Both CosmoDerm and CosmoPlast are FDA-approved human collagen fillers produced from purified human dermal cells and manufactured under strict environmental conditions. They can be used for reducing wrinkles and acne scars, for enhancing lips, and for reducing the signs of aging on the forehead, around the eyes and mouth, and in areas where collagen has diminished over time and facial contours have been lost.

As with other dermal fillers, the results are immediate and it can take as little as five minutes to achieve dramatic improvement. No pretreatment testing is required, unlike bovine collagen fillers, which require a skin test twenty-eight days before treatment.

CosmoDerm and CosmoPlast are injected below the surface of the skin using a very fine needle and there is very little, if any, discomfort. There is no downtime with these noninvasive procedures.

Most people ask how long the results will last, and the manufacturers of these products say that to maintain optimal correction, it is best to plan for minor touch-ups two or three times a year, although many people need them less often.

Evolence

Evolence is the newest FDA approved filler made of natural collagen that when injected, mimics your skin's own collagen allowing it to integrate beautifully and support your skin's existing collagen network. Evolence is typically used in moderate to deep facial wrinkles and folds such as the nasolabial folds. Like other fillers, there is no need for pre-testing, results are immediate, and there is no downtime. What makes Evolence different than other fillers is that the immediate results last much longer than the results from older types of collagen, and patients report less swelling and bruising after their treatment with Evolence than with other types of fillers.

Getting the Best Results from Dermal Fillers

If you want to get optimum results from your treatment, you can begin a regimen one week before the procedure by stopping the use of aspirin, certain anti-inflammatory medications, vitamin E, and fatty acids like Q10, flaxseed oil, and cod liver oil. Avoid high sodium, caffeine, and high sugar foods about two days before treatment. Two days after treatment, go back to your regular routine, remembering that caffeine, alcohol, smoking, and high sodium and high sugar are never good for you. This is a great time to give up bad habits and rethink your lifestyle.

The Best Treatment for You

Only your doctor can tell you which dermal fillers are best for your specific situation. (For information on choosing your doctor, see Chapter 16.) In some cases, a combination of products, together with Botox injections may be the right solution. This is a growing field with new products being approved on a regular basis for use in the United States. Even if you are currently having one kind of treatment, there is always the possibility that something new has been introduced since publication of this book. And remember, if you want to regain and retain the appearance of youth and vitality, dermal fillers are an ideal, safe, noninvasive alternative with no downtime.

CHAPTER 6

VolumaLift:

A Return to Youthfulness Without Surgery

With a VolumaLift (also known as the "Liquid Facelift"), there is now a way to address many of the problem areas that cause you to look in the mirror and shake your head at what you see. You know those areas: the hollows where you once had full cheeks, the sagging jawline, the sinking look of your eyes, and lines and furrows that have formed around your eyes and mouth.

If you are like most people, you have succumbed to the advertising for those "fountain of youth" cosmetic products. Beauty creams for day, intensive night products, lip treatments, and special eye gels. You have spent hundreds of dollars on these products after hearing the claims of firmer, lifted, plumper, younger-looking skin. And you have probably been disappointed with the results.

You have probably stood in front of that hateful mirror pulling your loose skin up and back and contemplating whether you are ready to go under the knife. You may even have gone to a cosmetic surgeon for a consultation and decided to wait. That is often code for "I am not sure that I am ready for something invasive and time consuming."

I know people like that.

"I'm 49 years old and stay in good shape. I eat right and exercise regularly, but I still look tired and old, and no amount of makeup can cover my wrinkles, fill in the hollows in my cheeks, or plump up my mouth and lips. I don't want to look unnaturally young—just fresher and brighter than I do now."

Donna C., age 49, Landscaper

"My mouth is already thin, but now it's sinking into deep lines and folds. I look like I am frowning all the time. I'm tired of people asking me what's wrong. Even though I am 60 years old, I want to look happy and young again."

Joanne W., age 60, Nurse

Now with VolumaLift, there is a wonderful, nonsurgical solution for people like Donna and Joanne and maybe for you as well. Best of all, the problem areas are all treated at one time in about half an hour or less.

Aging Causes the Problems

It may be a painful process, but this is a perfect time to pull out that old photo album and see how you have aged. You will be almost instantly aware of the full contours, tight jawline, full brows, plump lips and cheeks, and bright eyes of the youthful face. Now, hold up your favorite of these old photos next to your "today" face, and look at both in the mirror.

How did you get from that photo to the face you currently have? It didn't happen all at once. As you age, you lose important areas of facial fat known as buttresses, which support the contours of your face. First, you see the little crow's-feet and smile lines. Then your brow line begins to fall, your jaw line sags, and you lose the fullness in your cheeks, lips, and nose areas. To put it simply, you actually deflate and descend as you age.

In the past, traditional surgical facelifts were used to pull and tighten the skin but without replacing the fullness under the skin, the result can be a face that looks gaunt and hollow.

To get back that look of youth, you need to replace the support that you've lost. The VolumaLift does that quickly with minimal downtime and without surgery. It's not surprising that this procedure has become the procedure of choice for reshaping the face. Recently, *New York Magazine* reported that the "New *'New'* Face" is one that is "volumized" to re-create the soft, natural, youthful contours that help you look more like you did 10 years ago. It's no wonder many of today's celebrities are using this procedure to refresh their looks.

How VolumaLift Works

The VolumaLift uses injectable dermal fillers, such as Restylane, to restore volume and fullness. This miraculous product, a match for your own body's natural hyaluronic acid, which has been used for years to fill the lines and folds of the face, was the second most common cosmetic procedure (after Botox) in 2007.

When a VolumaLift is performed, the product is injected deeper into one or more of the buttresses of your face to instantly replace the volume that you have lost through aging. It can be used to plump up your eyebrows, fill in the hollows of your cheeks and lips, and contour your jawline to get back the lifted look of youth.

This is not a surgical procedure and there is no cutting involved, so there is no lengthy recuperation period. Unlike surgical facelifts that only pull and tighten your skin and sometimes make a deflated face look gaunter, a Voluma-Lift plumps up hollowed and sunken areas of your face. Also, because the dermal filler is placed deeper than when used only as wrinkle filler, the results of the procedure last longer.

Questions, Questions, Questions

The VolumaLift is relatively new, and most patients who come for a consultation ask the same questions. To make it easier for you to decide if this procedure is right for you, I have selected the most common questions to answer. This doesn't replace a session with your own doctor, however, so write down any others that are not answered here.

1. What areas of the face can benefit from a VolumaLift?

All areas including eyebrows and under the eyes, nasolabial areas, hollow cheeks, chin, lips, the upper lip area, and the sagging jawline can be treated. That includes virtually all six of the facial buttresses.

2. Is a VolumaLift safe?

Yes, the procedure has been tested and proven, and often uses the FDA-approved filler Restylane—the second most requested cosmetic product after Botox—which is completely compatible with your body's own hyaluronic acid, so allergy testing is not required.

3. How long does a VolumaLift last?

Everyone is different, of course, but since the dermal filler is placed deeper into the sunken and hollow areas of your skin, it can last much longer than when the filler is used in superficial wrinkles and lines. Today, there are new products being developed that last even longer than Restylane. Ask your doctor if they are available for your VolumaLift.

4. How long does a VolumaLift take?

It generally takes about thirty minutes, depending, of course, upon how many areas are treated.

5. Is the procedure painful?

Everyone is different, but most people say the Voluma-Lift procedure is generally not uncomfortable. The skin is frozen with local anesthesia before the procedure and the thin needles are passed through only the frozen skin. One interesting note is that treatment with injectable fillers can be more painful when injected into lines than when it is used in a VolumaLift. This is because there are very few pain fibers located very deeply along the facial bones, while there are more in the superficial areas.

6. How quickly will I see results?

Immediately. When the procedure is completed, you will see improvement in the shape and contours of your face. Some people can experience bruising and swelling, but this can be minimized with proper care. Always stop taking medically unnecessary aspirin, certain anti-inflammatory medications, and blood thinners about a week before the procedure.

7. Will I have any downtime?

Most people go back to their regular activities right away, but others are self-conscious about any bruises and swelling that might occur. A touch of makeup can help conceal any bruises that may be present after the VolumaLift treatment.

8. Are there alternatives to a VolumaLift?

There are some alternatives for volume restoration. These include fat injections using your own harvested fat. Voluma-Lift has been proven to be the least invasive option and very long lasting. Its results are also among the most effective, age appropriate ones available today.

9. Can I have this procedure with other procedures?

There are a number of procedures, including Botox, Thermage, Fraxel lasers, and photo facials that can be combined with a VolumaLift to help you achieve the specific results that you are seeking. Your doctor will work with you to determine if these should be done at the same time as a VolumaLift or at another time.

10. Can any doctor perform this procedure?

No. An injectable face-lift should be performed by a board certified cosmetic surgeon who has also been specifically trained and certified in the VolumaLift procedure.

11. How should I select the right doctor?

Always make sure that the doctor is qualified and certified to perform any procedure. Ask about how many procedures of this specific kind the doctor has done.

Understand his or her credentials and ask about special training in cosmetic procedures. Inquire about certification from boards and organizations recognized as leaders in the cosmetic field. Also, ask how often the doctor has performed a VolumaLift. If the doctor evades your questions or is not forthcoming, go somewhere else to have the procedure done. See Chapter 16 for more information on choosing your doctor.

12. How much does a VolumaLift cost?

As with any procedure of this type, cost varies depending on which areas are treated and how extensively. Your doctor should be able to tell you about your specific situation at a consultation.

Results

While everyone's expectations and results will be different, it is worthwhile to revisit both Donna and Joanne, the women who complained about their tired, aging experience.

"I looked tired and worn out before, but with the VolumaLift, I had immediate rewards. My face looks great and people can't believe how much younger and refreshed I look without surgery."

Donna C., age 49, Landscaper

"With a VolumaLift, my entire mouth and cheek area lifted and perked up. I'm amazed that such a simple procedure could make me look so much younger. I don't look frowny any more."

Joanne W., age 60, Nurse

What's Next

Evaluate your needs and ask your doctor if a VolumaLift might be right for your specific problems. It could be exactly the procedure you need to restore your youthful, refreshed appearance without surgery.

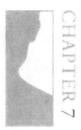

CHAPTER 7

Smartlipo MPX™ Laser Assisted Lipolysis:
Take Off What Dieting and Exercising Won't

No matter how strict their diet or how intense their exercise regimen is, there are many people who have areas of fat deposits that they cannot get rid of such as "love handles," double chins and saddle bags.

In the past, anyone hoping to remove stubborn fat deposits had only a couple of options that sometimes required lengthy treatment schedules to follow or traditional liposuction that required hospitalization, long downtime and long recovery periods and possible side effects from general anesthesia. If the area of fat to be removed was small, such as the ankle or the side of the knee, traditional liposuction could not be performed.

Now with Smartlipo MPX™ Laser Assisted Lipolysis, the next generation of minimally invasive laser sculpting treatments, patients can get rid of stubborn fat deposits and tighten skin for a smoother body shape. Not only is Smartlipo MPX effective in reshaping areas of the body and face, but it is less invasive than classic liposuction and delivers more immediate results with less downtime and side effects.

Smartlipo MPX Basics

Smartlipo was approved by the FDA in 2006 for its use as a laser liposculpting system. The Smartlipo MPX, the most technologically advanced Smartlipo system, uses two wave-lengths of laser light offering even better results than the original Smartlipo laser. Smartlipo MPX laser works by melting away fat and tightening skin in one treatment. The technology used in Smartlipo MPX dissolves fat more efficiently and with much less trauma to the body than traditional liposuction.

Smartlipo MPX is usually performed under local anesthesia and can be performed in an office setting. Offering significantly reduced and minimal downtime, patients treated with Smartlipo MPX can often return to work in a day or two versus one to two weeks with traditional liposuction.

One of the greatest benefits of Smartlipo MPX is its ability to tighten the skin so the patient is not left with sagging, loose skin after the fat is removed. The laser used in Smartlipo MPX also coagulates the blood vessels so that there is significantly less bruising and bleeding then with traditional liposuction, leading to an overall quicker recovery.

Almost anyone can be a good candidate for Smartlipo MPX. In general, ideal candidates are men and women who are not significantly overweight and who have only small areas of troublesome, localized fat deposits. Typical body areas treated include the "love handles," upper arms, neck and chin, abdomen, hips, buttocks, thighs, and knees.

How Smartlipo MPX Works

Smartlipo MPX uses a precise, safe and carefully calibrated laser-tipped cannula, or tube, approximately 1.0 millimeter in diameter. The laser is inserted just under the skin through a very small opening in the skin which does not need sutures and heals by itself, virtually disappearing in time. The small cannula delivers a series of rapid laser pulses that helps shrink the underside of the skin and selectively ruptures fat cells and liquefies fat deposits. The resulting oily, liquid substance is then gently removed. The small Smartlipo MPX laser also seals blood vessels as is zaps fat, so there is less bleeding, bruising and quicker recovery time than with traditional liposuction.

Given the cannula's small size and gentleness of the procedure, Smartlipo MPX laser-assisted lipolysis is a minimally invasive treatment that only requires local anesthesia with fewer side effects than traditional liposuction.

After the Smartlipo MPX treatment, an elastic compression garment may need to be worn in order to control and reduce swelling and help the body mold to its new shape. Many people often see an immediate improvement usually within a few days following their treatment with optimal results occurring three to six months later. Patients resume normal activities within one or two days of their treatment.

Questions, Questions, Questions

You probably have a great many questions about Smartlipo MPX. Here are some of the most often asked.

1. Which areas of the body can Smartlipo MPX be performed?

Smartlipo MPX has been designed to treat localized pockets of fat on the face and body. Typical areas include the chin and neck, upper arms, abdomen, "love handles," hips, buttocks, inner and outer thighs and knees. Your doctor can tell you if Smartlipo MPX is the right solution for your specific problem.

2. Does Smartlipo MPX treat cellulite?

The Smartlipo MPX procedure will improve the body's shape and may reduce cellulite to a certain degree.

3. Is Smartlipo MPX safe?

Yes. The laser method for fat removal and body sculpting has been used in Europe, Asia, and South America for about 10 years, and Smartlipo MPX was approved by the FDA for use in the United States in 2006. Your physician can tell you what to expect.

4. How long will the procedure take?

Since the treatment is personalized, only your physician can tell you how long a session will take. Generally, based upon the size of the treatment area, it can take from an hour to a few hours. It is performed in the doctor's office.

5. Does the Smartlipo MPX procedure hurt?

Since the Smartlipo MPX procedure is performed under local anesthesia, there is little pain or discomfort involved. Patients may feel an impression of tugging during the treatment, but this discomfort is minimal.

6. What side effects, if any, should I expect?

Most people experience minimal bruising and are pain free. Depending on the area treated, patients may need to wear a pressure dressing or compression garment. The mild ache is easily managed with oral pain medication. Typical bruising goes away over two to three days and patients can return to normal activities within twenty-four hours of their treatment.

7. Will I see results immediately?

Results are seen soon after the Smartlipo MPX procedure as the treated area will appear tighter, more compact, and smaller. It takes about six to eight weeks for the skin and surrounding area to remodel and adjust to the body contour. Remodeling is a gradual process with best results seen after two to three months.

8. What is the cost of having Smartlipo MPX done?

Cost depends upon which areas are treated and the size of the treatment area. Your physician is the most knowledgeable about this.

9. How do I select a doctor to perform Smartlipo MPX?

As with any medical procedure, it is important to understand your doctor's credentials and the experience that he or she has with a specific procedure. Look for a doctor that is board certified and has excellent certifications in Smartlipo MPX along with cosmetic treatments and procedures, look at before and after photos, and ask how often the doctor has performed Smartlipo MPX. Go with a doctor who can answer all of your questions to your satisfaction. See Chapter 16 for more information about choosing your doctor.

The Benefits of Smartlipo MPX

Following are some of the best benefits of Smartlipo MPX:

- Smartlipo MPX is minimally invasive with fewer side effects
- Smartlipo MPX is FDA approved for fat removal & body sculpting
- Smartlipo MPX involves use of a laser in the fat removal/sculpting process
- Smartlipo MPX is designed to treat localized pockets of fat in targeted areas
- Smartlipo MPX results can be seen after only one treatment
- Smartlipo MPX melts away as much as 3500 mls of fat in one session
- Smartlipo MPX treatments can be performed under local anesthesia
- Smartlipo MPX treatments cause less pain, less swelling & bruising
- Smartlipo MPX treatments are performed in the physician's office.

CHAPTER 8

Thermage:
Tissue Tightening that Works

Sagging skin is one of the most obvious signs of aging. It can show up on your face, upper arms, tummy, and other places, including your thighs and above the knees. It can even be the result of living a healthy life since weight loss is one of its causes.

Thermage, a nonsurgical skin tightening procedure, can successfully reduce the sagging problem and give the look of tighter, smoother skin from head to toe. It can even get rid of that "turkey neck"—that neck skin you pull back every time you look in the mirror at home. Because it is noninvasive, this procedure leaves no scarring, a problem with surgical alternatives. Who wants to solve one problem while possibly creating another?

Everyone has different reasons for having his or her skin tightened. Here are some examples of people who are looking for nonsurgical solutions specifically for facial problems:

"My face and neck are starting to sag and get looser, and I'm getting jowls and droopy eyelids. Help!"

Carol R., age 49, Warranty Administrator

"I'm too young for this. At 51, my eyelids are sagging so badly that the skin is nearly covering my eyes."

Holly D., age 51, Marketing Director

It's true that sagging skin makes us look older, less vibrant, and more tired than we want to look. Thermage delivers tighter skin, renewed facial contours, and increased collagen, the building block that provides structure to your skin. This treatment is only available from qualified physicians who specialize in cosmetic procedures.

Thermage Basics

Thermage is a noninvasive, nonsurgical treatment that tightens tissue by increasing collagen production. The doctor uses a patented technology called ThermaCool to tighten and gently lift skin to smooth out wrinkles and renew contours. The FDA has cleared the ThermaCool device for the noninvasive treatments of wrinkles and rhytids—the deep grooves in the skin that are caused by the skin's inability to maintain its strength and elasticity as a person grows older or deals with sun damage.

The procedure has been featured on *Oprah*, *The Today Show*, and in numerous media outlets as the "nonsurgical face-lift" and, unlike some lasers, can be performed on all skin types.

Since its introduction in 2002, Thermage has improved and refined its technology, now known as ThermaCool NXT, which allows the physician to easily target smaller and harder to handle problem areas. Thermage is no longer just an excellent non-surgical facelift, but can safely be used to improve the appearance of loose and sagging skin around the eye area, eyelids, face, neck and many parts of the body including the arms, abdomen, legs and buttocks. It also can reduce unwanted inches and the appearance of cellulite.

Thermage is a great solution if you are looking for natural improvement and skin rejuvenation; if health limitations, time, or cost affects your ability to have a surgical face-lift; or if you are simply not ready to go under the knife.

It can be used in combination with treatments such as Botox, dermal fillers, Mesotherapy/LipoDissolve, Smartlipo, and others, to meet your specific needs. A consultation with your cosmetic specialist is the best way to develop an individualized action plan.

How Thermage Works

Thermage uses radiofrequency (RF) technology to deliver a controlled amount of RF to uniformly heat a targeted area of collagen in the deeper layers of the skin's underlying tissue while simultaneously helping to protect the outer layer of the skin with cooling. This immediately tightens and lifts the skin to smooth out wrinkles and renew facial contours; it will tighten, firm, and shape the body while reducing the appearance of cellulite.

It is cosmetic science at its best, accomplishing what was only available from a surgical face-lift in the past. Unlike surgical procedures, there is no downtime. This gentler solution gives excellent results.

Questions, Questions, Questions

You probably have a great many questions about Thermage. Here are some of the most often asked.

1. Which areas of the face and body can Thermage tighten?

This is a very versatile procedure. It can be used on any area of the face, forehead, eyes, eyelids, neck, and chin where skin is sagging and needs to be tightened. In addition, there has been a great deal of success with upper arms, hands, upper legs, abdomen, and buttocks. Your doctor can tell you if Thermage is the right solution for your specific problem.

2. Is Thermage safe?

Yes. The Thermage procedure has been studied and is FDA approved. There have been more than 450,000 worldwide patient treatments with only a tiny incidence of side effects. These generally resolve in a few days or weeks. Some people experience a mild redness, similar to sunburn, but it usually disappears quickly. Your physician can tell you what to expect.

3. What does the Thermage procedure feel like?

With each touch of the Thermage device, you will experience a brief, deep-heating sensation as the RF energy is delivered to your skin and underlying tissue. This is your indication that your collagen is reaching an effective temperature for tightening. The device is cooled before, during, and after heating to protect your skin and make the treatment more comfortable. Many patients say that they experience a brief hot sensation followed by an immediate cool sensation. Your doctor should be able to ensure that you are comfortable and will sometimes apply an anesthetic cream to minimize any discomfort during the procedure.

4. How long will the procedure take?

Since the treatment is personalized, only your physician can tell you how long a session will take. Generally, based upon the size of the treatment area, it can take from a few minutes to an hour or so. It is usually performed in the doctor's office.

5. How many treatments will I need?

Unlike many laser procedures that require multiple sessions, a single Thermage treatment produces results in the majority of patients. That makes the procedure a cost-effective one when compared with some laser alternatives.

6. Will I see results immediately?

Immediately after you have a Thermage procedure done, you should feel a tightening and smoothing of your skin and a more youthful appearance. Everyone, of course, is unique, and the results are cumulative over several months' time.

7. How long will the results last?

The Thermage procedure causes immediate tightening of your collagen structure with additional tightening over time. Recent published studies conducted by Thermage show that measurable tightening improvements appear gradually over two to six months after a single treatment session. Everyone is different, of course, but depending upon your natural aging process, the results last a few years in most patients.

8. When can I resume my normal activities?

Immediately. There is no downtime and no special care required after a Thermage treatment. This is because it is a nonsurgical procedure.

9. What is the cost of having Thermage done?

Cost depends upon which areas are treated and the size of the treatment area. Your physician is the most knowledgeable about this. Ask beforehand what to expect.

10. How do I select a doctor to perform Thermage?

As with any medical procedure, it is important to understand your doctor's credentials and the experience that he or she has with a specific procedure. Look for someone with excellent certifications in Thermage along with cosmetic treatments and procedures, look at before and after photos, and ask how often the doctor has performed Thermage. Go with a doctor who can answer all of your questions to your satisfaction. See Chapter 16 for more information about choosing your doctor.

Results

Patients have great things to say after Thermage.

"After my full-face Thermage treatment, I was thrilled to see immediate results and my boyfriend noticed an amazing difference in less than twenty-four hours."

Carol R., age 49, Warranty Administrator

"I cancelled my surgical face-lift appointment after the awesome results I had with Thermage. I didn't need general anesthesia,

went directly from the doctor's office to an appointment, and taught an aerobics class the next morning. No one knew I had this treatment, but my husband and my mother both saw results quickly. I would recommend Thermage to anyone looking for a discrete approach to a more youthful appearance."

Holly D., age 51, Marketing Director

"Immediately after Thermage treatment for a brow lift, my friends complimented me on how my eyes looked bigger and brighter. It was thrilling to see results without undergoing general anesthesia."

Matthew R., age 46, Real Estate Agent

The Benefits of Thermage

Following are some of the best benefits of Thermage:
* Thermage is safe and effective
* Thermage is nonsurgical
* Thermage has no downtime
* Thermage has long-lasting results
* Thermage reduces wrinkles and smoothes out the skin
* Thermage safely reduces hooding, improves texture and tone, and softens fine lines and crow's feet in the eye area
* Thermage helps redefine facial and body contours
* Thermage lifts sagging skin on arms, legs, abdomen, and buttocks
* Thermage reduces unwanted bulges and smoothes the appearance of cellulite
* Thermage gives you natural-looking results without the pulled or stiff look sometimes associated with surgical procedures.

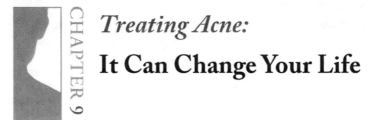

CHAPTER 9

Treating Acne:
It Can Change Your Life

Whether it is an active condition or one that has left you with scarring, acne is a serious affliction that can dramatically affect a person's life. Self-esteem is often sacrificed and research has shown that business success and relationships are often limited by people's perceptions. Bluntly put, no matter how terrific a person you are, the acne or scarring is what people see. Many who suffer from this condition say that looking in the mirror can be a painful experience, too.

A research study by one company that produces dermal fillers found that people with acne or post-acne skin problems tended to be introverted, held back in career and personal choices, covered their faces with their hair when they could, and generally avoided eye contact. Many of the study participants stated that they felt guilty about their condition although they knew that they had done nothing to cause it.

There was a time when the medical profession could offer little to a person suffering from acne or its aftermath. Today, there are many alternatives for both an active acne condition and for minimizing the appearance of scarring.

Acne Explained

Acne is the most common skin disease in the world. It not only troubles teenagers, but is a skin condition that also affects people of all ages. There are many people who are allergic to or experience side effects from the many medications that are used to treat acne. Fortunately, there are now new lasers and other treatments that can be used to improve acne and acne scarring.

There are many myths that surround acne. Among these are that blackheads are dirt, only teenagers have acne, certain foods like chocolate cause acne, and that acne will disappear on its own. In fact, the belief that untreated acne will disappear on its own is the cause of many people's scarring misery.

Acne occurs when the oil produced by sebaceous glands is trapped in the skin's tiny pores or follicles. When this oil plug closes off the pore, it can cause a whitehead, typically called a pimple. If the pore stays open, the top surface of the plug darkens, causing a blackhead. When either of these conditions occurs, it creates a place for the bacteria to thrive and spread. The pus and bacteria leak from the affected pore or follicle and affect the surrounding tissue, causing acne.

A person's teenage years are when acne first appears in most cases, but it can be a condition that continues or recurs at any age when a person is experiencing hormonal shifts that accompany the increase of oil. Some of the adult onset causes are menstrual periods, use of birth control pills, some oil-based products, and stress.

Different Levels of Acne Problems

Acne, as I have said, is caused by an oil plug in the skin's pores or follicles. The depth of the plug and the inflammation that surrounds it affects how bad the condition is. A plug that is close to the surface without much inflammation might cause a whitehead or blackhead, while one that is deeper in the follicle might cause a red bump or pustule.

Acne scarring is often caused when the oil plug forms deep within the follicle with a great deal of inflammation. In this case, a cyst forms and it is called cystic acne, which causes the scarring that is so traumatic.

Dermatologists classify acne into graded categories. Grade one is whiteheads and blackheads, which most people think of as teenage acne, although it can appear at any age. Grade two adds red bumps to the mix, but is still a manageable condition in most cases. The third grade begins deeper in the skin and has pustules that can cause scarring. It is the fourth grade—cystic acne—that most frequently causes scarring. Since the cysts begin deep within the skin and have a great deal of inflammation associated with them, they can do tremendous damage while they are active and result in extensive scarring even after the active condition is under control.

Treating Active Acne

Your doctor can easily determine the severity of an active acne problem and prescribe topical products, oral antibiotics, comedolytics such as Retin-A, sebostatics such as Accutane, and exfoliants, either separately or in combination.

All have the potential for side effects. However, newer acne treatments cause fewer of these undesirable problems. Ask your doctor about these recent advances:

- High-intensity blue light that specifically kills the bacteria responsible for acne vulgaris—the most pervasive form of acne

- Microdermabrasion with or without vitamin C (ascorbic acid)
- Photothermolysis laser treatments targeted to stimulate a photoactivated byproduct that kills acne-causing bacteria.

Solutions for Taming the Aftermath of Acne

Just as everyone is different, every case of acne or acne scarring is highly personal and requires personalized attention from your doctor. Most of the treatments mentioned briefly in this section are covered at greater length throughout this book. Following are some of the most frequent solutions for treating acne scarring:

- Dermal fillers treat shallow and deep acne scars. The procedure requires filling of shallow and deep acne scars, and improves the appearance of depressions. Results are immediate and patients generally require a touch-up every six months to two years, depending on which fillers are used.
- Dermabrasion works well on both raised and depressed areas of severe acne scars. The affected skin is treated with an anesthetic and the top dermal layer is then "sanded down" with a wire brush or diamond burr. Seven to ten days later, the skin forms a new, smoother layer. A full recovery can be expected in about six weeks.
- Microdermabrasion is done by using micro-crystals vacuumed over the skin's surface to remove damaged skin cells. The treatments are progressive and applied through a course of regular sessions. The "skin polishing" can provide a noticeable improvement to acne-scarred skin without discomfort. Your doctor can tell you how

many treatments will be needed to improve your specific condition.

- Chemical peels use chemical solutions available in several strengths to burn away the fine outer layers of skin. The strength of the solution used depends upon the degree of peeling necessary to rid you of the affected skin. Healing times are variable depending on the depth of the peel.

- Non-ablative laser and intense pulsed light (IPL) treatments are not painful and there is no downtime, making these very popular procedures for acne-scarred skin. Most patients receive a series of treatments, and, depending upon the type of acne scar, improvement can be dramatic. Continuing improvement is seen even after the treatments stop and results are cumulative.

- Laser resurfacing is a procedure that gently vaporizes the damaged or acne-scarred skin to reveal a new skin layer underneath. Depending upon the extent of the problem, laser scar removal is performed with local anesthesia for limited areas or with intravenous sedation by an anesthesiologist for a full-face treatment.

- Fractioned laser resurfacing (including the non-ablative Fraxel re:store and minimally ablative Fraxel re:pair) are the newest most advanced laser procedures that use a "fractional" approach to laser resurfacing with no downtime as compared to traditional fully ablative lasers. These newest lasers are able to target and treat only a fraction of the skin at a time so the surrounding untreated tissues help heal the skin much faster. The non-ablative Fraxel re:store Laser typically requires a series of treatments spaced three to four weeks apart. The fractionally ablative Fraxel re:pair Laser typically requires only one treatment performed under local anesthesia and has downtime typically of a few days. Your physician will help you decide which treatment is best for you depending on the extent of the problem.

Healing the Scars

While the scarring can be improved dramatically through these and the array of upcoming solutions that are being offered, it is also important to recognize that many of the scars caused by acne cannot be seen. It is true that the greatly improved appearance and the more favorable response of others to it are a great beginning. It is critical that you have realistic expectations. Don't expect your life to change overnight. After all, the acne problem didn't start yesterday. It became a problem over time and it will take time for you to see the complete results and the change that they will make in your life.

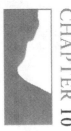

CHAPTER 10

In the Red:
Rosacea, Red or Brown Spots, and Other Vascular Problems

If your skin is reddish or appears flushed and blotchy, there are a number of causes. As with acne, this unattractive condition can affect your self-esteem and the perception of others. Some people, for example, mistake the connection between this flushed appearance and alcoholism, although too much alcohol can be a contributor.

The redness is generally caused by the dilation or expansion of tiny blood vessels. Often, people experiencing this problem have larger or more numerous blood vessels closer to the skin's surface. With repeated blushing, flushing, and sun damage, in addition to other normal responses, these blood vessels can become permanently dilated. Rosacea, which can appear with or without acne, is a vascular problem that is recurrent and often becomes permanent.

For decades, no one addressed this problem and it was treated more as an embarrassment than a skin disease. That has changed with the development of treatments and procedures that can minimize or eliminate the blotchy red skin conditions.

Recognizing Rosacea

Rosacea usually starts between the ages of thirty and fifty but the onset may be earlier or later. It is generally more common among fair-skinned people with a tendency to blush or flush easily. Certain lifestyles can make the condition worse, but they do not cause it. In fact, no one knows for sure what causes rosacea. At the beginning, it may appear to come and go without treatment. During its progression, it may include the center of the face, cheeks, forehead, chin, nose, and ears. Some cases also include the back and chest.

Often called "adult acne," rosacea pimples first appear as small reddish bumps. Then there is persistent redness of the face; once the problem reaches the state where the blood vessels never return to their normal appearance, it is time to ask the advice of a doctor.

Simply hoping that the condition will go away is not enough. Once rosacea reaches this stage, the only way to reverse it is to have effective treatment and change any of the factors that can make the problem worse.

Perhaps you have seen a person with a red bulbous nose and puffy red cheeks. This is an advanced rosacea condition called rhinophyma. (The typical image of Santa Clause might be a good example.)

There are a number of ways to minimize the effects of rosacea and, when combined with the right medical treatment, the appearance of rosacea can be effectively reduced. The following tips are based on conventional wisdom and common sense:

- Rosacea can be affected by hot drinks, spicy foods, caffeine, alcohol, and hormonal changes. If you are using hormone replacement therapy, try taking estrogen at night instead of in the morning. Avoiding these things can help to prevent outbreaks and keep reddening to a minimum.

- Always use good sun protection. It has been shown that sun exposure can make rosacea worse and, since it also causes premature skin aging, a smart approach that utilizes cover-ups, hats, and sunscreen should be followed.
- Temperature extremes have been shown to make rosacea and other reddening conditions worse. Try to avoid extreme cold and heat and, if you are prone to reddening, be sure to exercise in a cool environment and stop when you feel the flushing get worse.
- Don't rub and scrub or massage the face if you have a tendency toward redness or rosacea. It can irritate the skin.
- Avoid cosmetics and facial products that cause any irritation. Many over-the-counter skin creams and wrinkle products inflame the skin and aren't effective anyway. Keep hair spray away from your face.
- If you do have flushing and blushing episodes, keep a diary of foods, activities, products, and medications that may trigger them. It will help you to make lifestyle modifications once your rosacea is under control.

Treating Rosacea

Your doctor is, as always, the best source for medical solutions for skin problems. He or she can identify the problem and make the best recommendation for treating it depending upon the severity of the problem. In a number of cases, he or she may recommend more than one treatment including medications, lasers, and light therapies such as intense pulsed light (IPL) photorejuvenation.

Brown Spots and Patches

Brown spots can be caused by many things and may be due to aging, freckling, or melasma, a condition that becomes common with pregnancy or hormonal changes. Since natural light stimulates this condition, the best ways to avoid these annoying problems are to stay out of direct sunlight, to use a high-SPF sunscreen, and to cover up when you are outdoors.

Fortunately, with advances in technology there are a few treatments to treat brown spotting and patches including IPL and Fraxel re:store Laser to minimize or remove this discoloration. Only a consultation with your doctor can tell you which solution is right for your specific situation.

Intense Pulsed Light (IPL)

IPL is also known as photo-facial, fotofacial, and photo rejuvenation. This noninvasive, no downtime treatment is multifunctional. In addition to reducing the redness of rosacea and broken capillaries (those red veins that often appear around your nose and on your cheeks as you age, which are technically called telangiectases), IPL is also used to remove sun damage and some pigmented birthmarks that are caused by vascular issues. It is also used for hair reduction and some other conditions.

A highly advanced computer regulates a light pulse to a specific wavelength range that treats a portion of the affected skin. This minimizes the appearance of the damaged tissue, while avoiding contact with the surrounding skin. With IPL rejuvenation, the light pulses are directed at the blood vessels, age spots, freckles, flat, pigmented birthmarks, and rosacea.

Depending upon the wavelength used, the targeted tissues are either red blood cells in the dermis or melanin pigment in the uppermost skin layer. An additional bonus is that the treatment may stimulate tiny blood vessels to encourage the production of new collagen and further improve skin tone and texture.

IPL can also be used to reduce pore size and shrink oil glands, making this a good treatment option to combat acne and similar conditions.

Best Possible Candidates for IPL

As discussed earlier, men and women of all ages can consider this treatment for various skin problems, including:

- Brown or age spots
- Facial spider veins
- Rosacea
- Undesirable skin pigmentation
- Freckles
- Reducing pore size
- Shrinking enlarged oil glands

IPL treatments may not be the best treatments for you if you are dark skinned or darkly tanned or if you have inconsistent levels of skin pigmentation. If any of these are the case, your doctor may be able to offer other effective alternatives.

Advantages of IPL

The treatment is gentle in the hands of an experienced medical professional. There is no interruption of routine activities and no recovery time is needed. Since IPL is completely noninvasive, there are no stitches, cuts, or bleeding to be concerned with.

You will usually notice an improvement after one or two treatments, depending on the nature of your problem. Improvement is gradual and your doctor can tell you how many treatments you will need. Treatments can generally be given two to four weeks apart, upon the recommendation of your doctor.

Fraxel re:store Laser

Fraxel re:store Laser treatment is one of the most advanced breakthroughs in nonsurgical treatments available today. Fraxel re:store is FDA approved for skin resurfacing and the treatment of uneven skin pigmentation including brown spots and melasma, fine lines and wrinkles, and acne and acne scarring (as discussed in chapter 9).

In the past, anyone needing skin resurfacing had only a few "ablative" or "non-ablative" treatment options. The older fully ablative treatments such as CO_2 lasers destroy the surface of the skin and, while effective, they have a high probability of significant risks and long painful recovery times. "Nonablative" treatments did not remove the outer layer of skin and were gentler on your skin, but often only offered limited results.

With recent breakthroughs in laser technology, Fraxel re:store has become the gold standard in nonablative fractional resurfacing. It is designed to target and treat aging and damaged skin by treating portions of specific damaged tissues without affecting untargeted surrounding tissues. This fractional treatment targets 20-25% of the skin's surface at a time triggering your body's natural healing process and accelerating the production of collagen and new, healthy skin.

This new generation, nonsurgical treatment can be used on the face and body including the very delicate areas of the neck, eyes, chest and hands. And unlike some lasers, Fraxel re:store can be used on patients of all skin types.

Each Fraxel re:store treatment targets a percentage of your skin at a time so a series of four treatments spaced three to four weeks apart is ideal. Many patients notice improvement after the first treatment with most noticeable results after the third of fourth treatment. Side effects may include mild swelling and redness which usually resolve within a day or two after the treatment so you can return to your normal activities right away.

Some Afterthoughts

It is important to stay out of the sun and always use sunscreen. Be gentle with your skin and avoid scrubs, exfoliants, and alpha- or beta-hydroxyl acid products. Also, it is best to avoid excessive heat exposure such as saunas, steam rooms, hot showers, or baths for about twenty-four hours after a treatment.

As with any medical procedure of this type, your doctor will be able to guide you through your preparation and post care. See Chapter 16 for more information on selecting the best doctor for your treatment.

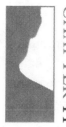

CHAPTER 11

Too Much of a Good Thing:
Laser Hair Removal

If someone were to ask me what is the most frequently performed cosmetic skin procedure, the answer is a simple one. More people in the United States and around the world have laser hair removal done than any other cosmetic laser treatment.

Attitudes about hair in different cultures are diverse but in Western and Asian cultures, particularly, most people prefer the appearance of a smooth, hairless body. While dealing with unwanted hair has always been a drag, laser hair removal has made the reduction of hair and the accompanying maintenance easy and convenient.

Where Hair Comes From

As babies, we are covered with a soft down of vellus hairs. This soft pale hair is everywhere, but as we grow older, our follicles produce thicker longer hairs in some parts of the body.

Puberty, for example, signals the growth of hair in areas that were once hairless, representing the increase of certain hormones. Menopause is reflected in a diminishing of hair as the growth recedes in many areas and becomes lighter and less dense.

This does not assure that the hair we have is necessarily in the areas that we want and shifting hormones—particularly in menopause—often cause women to have darker, coarser hair in undesirable places. It is also important to note that hair on the face grows faster than on other body areas.

The Causes of Unwanted Hair

As with so many conditions, unusual amounts of hair and hair in unwanted places are often due to a hereditary predisposition. Chances are that if your family has a history of dark, coarse hair on the arms, face, abdomen, chin, sideburn area, around the nipples, or on the abdomen or back, you will encounter the same condition.

There are other causes, of course, including polycystic ovary syndrome (a hereditary condition that affects the normal production of eggs because of cysts), which causes unwanted hair growth related to the additional circulation of typical male hormones. (Acne is also sometimes attributable to polycystic ovary syndrome.)

And it bears repeating that most cases of unwanted hair that are not hereditary are the result of hormonal cycles that occur throughout our teenage and adult lives. Interestingly, as our body signals for this thicker, darker hair as we age, the hair at our temples begins to recede and, particularly in women, the hair in the armpit and pubic areas also get sparser.

The Best Way to Get Rid of Unwanted Hair

Most people—other than those with extensive conditions—begin by trying to remove the unwanted hair at home. Plucking doesn't make the hair grow back thicker and longer. That is an "old wives'" tale. When you have one or two random hairs, this may be a solution, but if you are like many people, this isn't a good long-term solution. Neither are over-the-counter hair removal creams, which can be irritating to many people and often have an unpleasant smell.

Waxing can be costly and painful, especially for some tender body areas. Also, some people have difficulty with ingrown hairs, irritation, and the temperature to which the wax is heated for it to be effective. Shaving needs to be annoyingly frequent and razor blades can collect bacteria that can infect hair follicles and cause irritation.

Electrolysis treats only one hair follicle at a time, so it is impractical for larger areas of unwanted hair. That makes it practical only for those very small areas that are just as easily plucked. It is a lot of work to find a conveniently located, licensed, and experienced electrologist. Even then, if your time is limited, this is probably not the best solution for you. It can also be painful since an electrical current is passed down through a tiny wire to each follicle that is treated.

The best way to reduce unwanted hair—whether the condition is large or small—is with laser hair removal. This well-respected medical treatment can address virtually every case in which unwanted hair is a problem and, with regular maintenance, you can avoid dealing with the less comfortable and less reliable alternatives.

How Laser Hair Removal Works

When a medical professional performs laser hair removal, a specialized beam of light targets the pigment, which gives color to our skin and hair. Virtually any kind of skin is fine for this procedure, but hair that is darker, particularly on lighter skin, is easiest to deal with because all of the energy from the laser beam is absorbed by the hair follicle rather than the hair and the skin around it. This makes laser hair removal perfect for those wayward hairs and for treating larger areas. A highly trained medical professional with extraordinary expertise can treat dark hair on dark skin, but you need to be certain that this is within the doctor's range of knowledge and that a special type of laser is used if this is your problem.

Questions, Questions, Questions

You probably have questions about laser hair removal. Here are some of the most often asked.

1. Does the hair grow back?

Laser hair removal destroys hair follicles that are actively producing hair at the time of treatment. Hair follicles are not adequately destroyed when they are dormant or not producing hair. If dormant follicles are stimulated to produce hair by certain hormones (for example, during puberty), then new hairs will grow. Maintenance can be done when these new hairs grow.

It is good to know that with laser hair removal, to the exception of the other treatments commonly in use today, the laser does gradually reduce the number of hairs that grow back and, in most cases, the hair that does grow back is lighter and finer than what was originally treated. The effects of laser hair removal are cumulative.

2. Who should do my laser hair removal?

While this is a state-regulated field, it is important to understand that this medical procedure should be done under the supervision of a doctor. There can be serious complications including discoloration and scarring from a bad practitioner.

Your safety is the most important concern. This is not simply a matter of cosmetic care. Pick your doctor accordingly. See Chapter 16 for more information on choosing your doctor.

3. How often will I need maintenance?

As with most procedures, this is very subjective. Many patients say that their expectations are met with three to six treatments, while others say they are satisfied with more or fewer. Since laser hair removal needs to be done only when you feel that you need a touch-up (after having the initial treatments to reach your goal), it is up to you. You may find that you have hormonal flare-ups that require additional maintenance but if you follow a regular regimen, maintaining your desired appearance should be easy.

4. How long do treatments take?

Depending upon the size of the area being addressed, treatments can take several minutes to several hours. For larger areas, your doctor may recommend a series of treatments to make the time commitment easily manageable for you. Your doctor can tell you how long a treatment is expected to take, and since this is an entirely noninvasive procedure, there should be no downtime afterward. You can go back to your regular routine immediately.

5. How do I get ready for laser hair removal?

While you should always consult your doctor regarding your specific situation, the following are some recommended steps:

- For best results, don't do any procedures for hair removal—including plucking, bleaching, and electrolysis—for three or four weeks before your facial laser hair removal session and for up to eight weeks prior to laser hair removal on the body.
- It is okay to shave right up to the laser hair removal procedure.
- Don't tan or use self-tanners for at least two weeks prior to your treatment.
- Tell your doctor about any medications that you are taking or any problems that you may have had with hair removal alternatives in the past.

Following these tips will allow the unwanted hair follicles to be highly sensitive and should help to enhance your results. As with any medical procedure, ask your doctor for answers to your specific questions. As it has always been said, there is no such thing as a bad or silly question.

CHAPTER 12

Smoothing the Rough Edges:

Chemical Peels, Microdermabrasion and GentleWaves

Close your eyes and run your hand along the inside of your arm up to the elbow. That is the closest that most of us come to retaining the smooth skin of our youth. That skin has not been constantly exposed to weather, stress, and other conditions that affect appearance and texture. For most of us, that skin feels amazing.

If it were possible, who would decline the opportunity to regain that smooth skin on our faces and other parts of our bodies—free of fine lines; lack of sagging skin, scarring, and dark spots; sun damage; and a wide variety of other imperfections? Not many.

Today, it is possible through sophisticated procedures, products, and technology to do just that. Underneath the surface of the skin lies the unrevealed potential for that kind of appearance and texture.

A highly trained and experienced doctor can recommend the right approach for your specific problems and help to release the beautiful layer of skin that otherwise lies hidden.

Whether the recommendation is for a chemical peel, microdermabrasion, or GentleWaves LED Photomodulation (alone or in combination with other treatments and procedures), the exceptional results can be dramatic, like no other solution.

Multiple alternatives share the same objective, although one is sometimes favored over another for specific conditions. In the case of chemicals peels and microdermabrasions, damaged and worn tissue is exfoliated to remove the dull surface layer to reveal fresher skin. The level of penetration can also have an effect on reducing lines and wrinkles and encouraging the growth of new collagen. In the case of GentleWaves, a light source gently activates the skin's natural rejuvenation process from the inside out.

These are not your average fluff and buff spa treatment. Aesthetic technicians in spas in many states are not permitted to give many of these treatments and procedures. Only a doctor can make the appropriate recommendations and provide some of these services.

Chemical Peels

While chemical peels are not new, the ability to use them in a highly personalized manner to solve individual problems has been refined and improved over the past twenty years. This very popular alternative can be highly personalized to meet specific needs for treating the skin from surface to deep.

A light peel treats the surface level of the skin. It generally does not treat deep wrinkles, but is effective for removing the uppermost layer of dead skin cells for a fresh, revitalized appearance. Generally requiring less than an hour, the results can last for months if you stay out of the sun and maintain a desirable level of maintenance with light cleansers and moisturizers.

The doctor will probably use a mild glycolic or fruit acid and will encourage you to have a series of light peels for best results—more frequently at first, with greater spacing between treatments as the series progresses.

The next step up is a light-to-medium peel, which utilizes a stronger chemical solution and goes deeper into the dermis to treat sun damage, dark spotting, acne, or skin discoloration. This peel provides longer-lasting results, as do the more intense procedures that go deeper into the layers of the skin. In addition to the face, a light-to-medium peel is often done on other exposed areas of the body that exhibit similar damage.

A medium chemical peel offers even greater results and begins to address the targets of the lighter peels, while encouraging the growth of new collagen for a more youthful appearance. Fine lines begin to disappear and skin tone and texture improve. With regular treatments, given in a series, increased collagen makes skin firmer. The results of a series of medium-level chemical peels can last up to a few years.

Because of their effectiveness, medium peels are often done in conjunction with surgical and nonsurgical face-lifts to improve the condition of the skin, but it is wise to start a regimen before other alternatives to determine whether you need another procedure at all.

Deep peels are the strongest form of chemical peels and are prescribed only in the most severe cases. A deep peel is for medical conditions rather than rejuvenation and, if it is required, your doctor will thoroughly detail the procedure for you.

For most people, a medium peel provides everything that is both needed and desired for a newer, fresher appearance.

There are some guidelines to follow if you want to get the best results from your chemical peel:

- If you are a smoker, stop or cut back dramatically—this is a great time to quit. Cells regenerate faster if they aren't fighting the effect of smoking, which depletes oxygen.
- If your diet permits, add more protein for at least a few weeks before your peel. It is a nutritional addition that can add to your results.
- If you have a history of cold sores, be sure to let your doctor know. He may choose to give you medication to take before or after the treatment to prevent an outbreak.
- Stay out of the sun, wear sunscreen, and follow your doctor's maintenance instructions for the best outcome.

Microdermabrasion

For improving skin texture and color and tired-looking skin, microdermabrasion offers a gentle solution. The procedure utilizes micro-crystals that help to exfoliate the skin's surface when combined with a vacuuming that removes the dead cells and flakes that are hiding your skin's real beauty. Sometimes microdermabrasion is called "mini-sanding" but describing it as skin polishing is probably a better way to explain it.

Consider this: when a rough gem is mined from the earth, it often goes through a process that uses fine grit to polish it so that the inner glow is revealed. Microdermabrasion uses fine crystals to do the same thing.

This is an anti-aging treatment that can be used separately or in combination with other rejuvenating procedures such as chemical peels, injectables, Botox, and laser treatments.

Microdermabrasion can remove superficial brown spots and freckles, as well, but the results are usually not permanent. It is not the ideal solution for wrinkles, since there is so much technology that is dedicated only to minimizing lines and wrinkles.

Microdermabrasion is also an effective tool for minimizing the appearance of comedone (plugged pore) acne since it removes the upper layer of skin where the problems reside, and improves circulation to the skin.

As with chemical peels and many other anti-aging solutions, multiple treatments are often recommended for the best possible results. Ask your doctor to help develop a treatment plan that works for you, and follow his or her guidelines for maintaining your rejuvenated skin once you have begun your regimen.

GentleWaves LED Photomodulation

GentleWaves LED Photomodulation is a safe, simple anti-aging treatment that activates the skin's natural rejuvenation process, reducing wrinkles and improving skin tone and texture from the inside out for strong, smoother, radiant skin.

GentleWaves uses a carefully timed sequence of light emitting diodes (LEDs) that actually stops the production of enzymes that breakdown the collagen under your skin while simultaneously stimulating your skin's cells to produce collagen and elastin. This unique combination strengthens the skin's foundation and minimizes further breakdown.

GentleWaves is not a laser so it doesn't use heat. It is safe for all skin types. There is no pain, redness, peeling or other side effects or downtime. The treatments are quick, usually lasting about only a few minutes. This procedure has clinically demonstrated to show improvements in the majority of patients after eight treatments.

Due to its unique light source technology, GentleWaves can help maintain and possibly improve the results of many other cosmetic treatments including microdermabrasion, chemical peels, Botox, IPL and Fraxel laser treatments.

CHAPTER 13

Softening Lines and Wrinkles:
Pulsed Dye Laser Wrinkle Reduction

Just as lasers have changed the entire face of cosmetic rejuvenation, they can do the same for you. Fine wrinkles that age you and make you look tired or stressed are a perfect target. You needn't be old or feel old to gain the benefit of this noninvasive, pain-free procedure that enables your body to produce more collagen while improving the texture and polish of your skin. No needles are used and there is no downtime.

Pulsed dye laser wrinkle reduction uses gentle waves to reduce the facial wrinkles that make you self-conscious, but there is the added benefit of using laser technology to deal with other flaws at the same time. Redness and brown spotting from aging and sun damage can be addressed. Broken blood vessels and rosacea can be successfully treated. These are all accomplished using the precision control of the laser, which can target specific areas or be an extraordinary tool for an entirely fresh face.

The treatment is easy. Before the laser procedure, all your makeup is removed and the area that is to be treated is cleaned. During your treatment, the light energy from the laser is passed through a tool that allows your doctor to control the specific amount of energy needed to correct the problem area. You may experience slight warmth when the laser is used, but most people report little or no discomfort.

Improvement is gradual since your body requires time to produce the added collagen and for the wrinkles, lines, and other flaws to be diminished. Depending upon how much work is needed, several short office visits might be required.

Questions, Questions, Questions

There are some commonly asked questions regarding laser wrinkle and line reduction, as there are with most rejuvenation procedures. Here are some of the major ones.

1. I am seeing advertising for all kinds of laser and rejuvenation centers in my area. How do I know where I will get the best professional treatment?

Look specifically for a laser center associated with a doctor who is well known in your area for this type of procedure. You will always get the best results from a doctor who does a great many laser procedures. Avoid laser centers that are attached to many spa locations where the medical director may not be there much of the time. Look for an operation that has "laser" in its name and does not simply specialize in hair removal. Your care and results will generally be better with a doctor who dedicates a significant amount of time to laser procedures. (For more detailed information on selecting your doctor, see Chapter 16.)

2. I have found that estimates of cost for pulsed dye laser wrinkle reduction are all over the place. How do I know that I am not getting a bargain because the facility is not the most capable?

As with any true medical procedure, this is not the place for bargain shopping. The best laser surgeons are the ones who usually charge rates from the average to the higher end of the cost range. There are good reasons for this, one of which should not be ignored: First, they are usually better with this type of procedure. Second, they are busier because they are better. Third, the best equipment and continuing education are expensive, but you want them to incur that kind of expense even though it will be reflected in the costs. And, last, you want to know that all of the personnel in the office are the best in the field.

3. How long will my treatment take?

The length of treatment varies from a few minutes to an hour or more, depending on what areas need to be treated. Since it is noninvasive, you will have no downtime and can make plans directly afterward.

4. What kind of maintenance will be required?

Virtually every rejuvenation treatment or procedure requires some maintenance, even surgical ones. Nothing lasts forever in this field, but the results are worth it. You are continuing to age, even after the treatments; sun and smoking damage will still be a concern, along with spotting and other flaws. Your doctor can give you a good idea of what to expect and how long the results generally last. Remember, however, that your problems, skin type, and other conditions make the maintenance plan specific to you. Beware of any laser facility that promises you the moon in only one short treatment. You may be disappointed with the long-term results.

5. What should I do before I have my treatments?

You should do several things before you start your treatments:

- Ask questions. Make a list of your concerns and the problems that need to be dealt with before your consultation so you don't forget anything.
- Let the doctor tell you about any other flaws or conditions that he or she feels can be addressed during your course of treatment. They are the professionals for a reason.
- Pay full attention to pretreatment instructions and post-treatment responsibilities. The instructions are being provided to you for a reason. They are not hard to follow, nor are they demanding, and they may have a major effect on the results.

6. I have very deep wrinkles and lines. Can laser rejuvenation help my problem?

While deep wrinkles and lines are not the best targets for laser rejuvenation, a doctor who specializes in laser therapies can make recommendations for you as to other alternatives that might be better. That doctor is still your first step, no matter what.

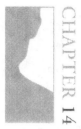

CHAPTER 14

Fraxel Laser Treatments:
Fractioned Skin Resurfacing and Tightening

Many patients have asked if there is a "magic wand" that can simply be waved over their face and body that can instantly make them look 10 years younger. Here is what a few patients had to say about their looks:

"I am 57 year-old successful retail manager. I have 3 grown children and one grandchild. In my youth I never used sun block and now I look so old! My skin looks like a comfortable old chair with wrinkles and splotches of dark skin. I just want my skin to look healthy again"

-Linda S., age 57

"I take better care of myself now as a 50-year-old than I did when I was 30, but my face didn't look it. I had brown spots from my sun-worshipping days and the crow's feet around my eyes became permanent."

-Eileen P., age 50

"After neglecting my skin and with sun and smoking damage, my face had aged considerably!"

-Mary W., age 60

Fraxel Laser Treatments are perhaps the closest we can come to a "magic wand." Fraxel Laser Treatments, known as Fraxel re:store and Fraxel re:pair, rejuvenate the skin, fix years worth of aging and sun damage, erase fine lines and wrinkles, get rid of acne and acne scarring and bring back soft, smooth, tighter skin that looks years younger.

Fraxel re:store Laser Treatments

Fraxel re:store Laser treatment is one of the most advanced breakthrough skin resurfacing treatments available today.

In the past, anyone needing skin resurfacing had only a few "ablative" or "non-ablative" treatment options. The older, fully "ablative" treatments destroyed the surface of the skin and, while effective, they have a high probability of significant risks and long painful recovery time. "Non-ablative" treatments did not remove the outer layer of skin and were gentler on your skin, but often did not offer the dramatically smooth results as were expected.

Fraxel re:store Laser treatment offers the same results of older, fully ablative treatments without the long recovery time.

Fraxel re:store is FDA approved for skin resurfacing including the treatment of fine lines and wrinkles, acne and acne scarring, and uneven skin pigmentation including brown spots and melasma.

This new-generation, nonsurgical treatment can be used on the face and body including the very delicate areas of the neck, eyes, chest and hands.

How Fraxel re:store Works

Fraxel re:store Laser treatment is designed to target and treat aging and damaged skin by targeting portions of specific damaged tissue.

To appreciate how Fraxel re:store works, think of a family portrait or digital photograph in need of high quality restoration or touch up. Just as a damaged painting is delicately restored one area at a time, or a photographic image is altered pixel by pixel, the Fraxel re:store Laser improves your appearance by affecting only a fraction of your skin at a time with thousands of microscopic laser spots. It's like photo-editing software for your skin.

The microscopic laser spots penetrate deep into the skin without affecting untargeted surrounding tissues. For every area the laser targets and treats intensively, it leaves the surrounding tissue unaffected and intact. This fractional treatment, meaning that it targets 20-25% of the skin's surface at a time, triggers your body's natural healing process accelerating the production of collagen and new, healthy skin.

Most patients experience immediate results and see the most benefit in three to five treatments spaced three to four weeks apart depending on their condition

Fraxel re:pair Laser Treatments

Fraxel re:pair Laser treatment is the long awaited newest addition to the Fraxel™ line of lasers. Now with Fraxel re:pair Laser you can have the dramatic results of a fractional ablative skin resurfacing combined with the tightening results of a facelift without the prolonged downtime and side effects associated with conventional fully ablative resurfacing lasers and surgical procedures. This treatment corrects severe skin damage while tightening the skin. Men and women are using Fraxel re:pair to postpone or eliminate the need for a surgical facelift.

This new groundbreaking laser treatment is the first fractionated CO2 laser to receive FDA clearance for skin resurfacing and the treatment of wrinkles, textural irregularities, and pigmentation including age spots, sunspots, and sun induced redness.

How Fraxel re:pair Works

Fraxel re:pair Laser is the first and only laser that addresses skin tightening and pigmentation all in one treatment. Fraxel re:pair uses a high intensity carbon dioxide laser to vaporize unwanted tissue using fractional technology which can achieve dramatic improvements similar to traditional bulk ablative CO2 treatments with considerably less downtime and risks.

Fraxel re:pair distinguishes itself by its ability to remove microscopic amounts of tissue deep in the skin, surrounded by undamaged healthy tissue. This stimulates the production of new collagen which tightens and smoothes the skin for a younger, healthier appearance. Most patients see improvement right away in a single treatment with ultimate results usually seen within three to six months.

The difference between
Fraxel re:store and Fraxel re:pair

Both Fraxel re:store and Fraxel re:pair lasers use Fraxel technology but in different ways. Fraxel re:store is a non-ablative technique that intensively treats older skin cells while leaving the skin's protective barrier intact. Fraxel re:pair is an ablative procedure that uses a carbon dioxide laser to vaporize microscopic tissue deep within the skin and stimulate collagen growth. Since Fraxel re:pair intensely treats the most severe skin damage, results are achieved in a single treatment and recovery may take a few days.

Benefits of Fraxel re:store and Fraxel re:pair Laser Treatments

- Fraxel lasers are safe, effective, and FDA approved
- Fraxel lasers treat multiple skin conditions and all skin types
- Fraxel lasers are the new way to restore and repair damaged facial skin
- Fraxel lasers are more effective and less invasive than older laser treatments
- Fraxel lasers can have the same results as older CO_2 and Erbium lasers without the downtime
- Fraxel lasers improve without lengthy downtime and fewer side effects
- Fraxel lasers encourage your body's own natural healing
- Fraxel lasers give you healthy beautiful skin by replacing damaged skin
- Fraxel lasers treat eye wrinkles, pigmented lesions, age spots, and sun spots
- Fraxel laser are the most advanced breakthrough available today in laser resurfacing
- Fraxel lasers are the new industry standard for aesthetic laser skin treatment.

Now here is what the patients you read about earlier had to say after their own Fraxel Laser treatment:

"I can't believe the results! After my Fraxel treatment my skin feels smoother and the brown spots are gone! My skin looks fresh

and healthy. The comments I get from people when they find out how old I am just make my day. Thank you!"

-Linda S., age 57

"*Fraxel made the brown spots and wrinkles on my face disappear! My skin is the smoothest that it has ever been.*"

-Eileen P., age 50

"*I can't say enough about this wonderful new fractional CO2 treatment. Immediately after my procedure I looked at least 10 years younger. This is such an incredible breakthrough. The procedure took maybe 30 minutes and with minimal discomfort only I went home, had no pain whatsoever. I was able to attend a wedding 4 days later! Dr. Covey took me one step at a time and his staff were so caring and supportive. I would never have anything done elsewhere. This is truly a gift in life – I feel younger and lighter!*"

-Mary W., age 60

The revolutionary lines of Fraxel Laser treatments are the most advanced tool you can use to reduce the signs of aging and give you back the beautiful, glowing skin that reflects the youth and vitality you feel inside.

CHAPTER 15

Mesotherapy and Lipodissolve:
Contouring Without Surgery

If you have ever pulled at a love handle, resented the jiggle of your inner thighs, or looked at your jawline or under your chin and said, "I would do anything short of surgery to get rid of this," then you may want to explore mesotherapy and lipodissolve as nonsurgical alternatives that create contours and reduce fat.

These are the kinds of problems that patients believe are critical to their well-being, appearance, and their confidence in themselves. Most of those who explore these alternatives said that they are not ready to see a plastic surgeon but that they are willing to undertake virtually any nonsurgical solution that offers results.

Following are some examples of problems that can be solved with mesotherapy and lipodissolve.

"I always had a problem with love handles. My jeans pushed all my fat into my middle."

Diane G., age 49, Real Estate Agent

"My problem areas included my hips and thighs, and I felt that my body was disproportionate."

Jennifer B., age 35, Retail Manager

"No matter how much I exercised or how much weight I lost, I still had bulges of fat on my upper thighs."

Marie C., age 48, Receptionist

"As I aged, my jaw line and the area under my chin were not firm and they pulled my face down. I thought that nothing short of surgery would solve the problem."

Linda R., age 60, PR Consultant

Mesotherapy and lipodissolve are not new procedures. As with many nonsurgical solutions, they were developed in Europe. French doctor Michel Pistor used the process as early as 1952. Today, they are done by certified medical practitioners around the world.

They do what no weight loss products, diets and exercise programs, or skin-firming lotions can do. Mesotherapy and lipodissolve can literally melt away fat and get rid of ugly cellulite in specific facial and body areas without surgery. And while it sounds too good to be true, the tens of thousands of people who have chosen to have the procedures are a perfect benchmark of success.

Mesotherapy and Lipodissolve Basics

Mesotherapy—the term comes from the Greek words for "middle" and "to treat medically"—is a procedure that stimulates the repair of tissues in the middle layer (or mesoderm) of the skin, connective tissue, and fat. The procedure is regularly used in Europe to treat various conditions, from sports injuries to chronic pain. It is so successful at treating a variety of problems, including cosmetic problems, that it has been featured on *CBS News*, *48 Hours*, *20/20*, *ABC News*, and in *People* magazine, *Elle*, and other media outlets.

Mesotherapy can be done on just about any part of your body. On the face, mesotherapy is excellent for the reduction of fat bags under the eyes, as well as the fat under the chin and around the jowls. It is also exceptional at reducing "love handles," as well as numerous areas of the body that do not respond to diet or exercise. Unlike liposuction, it can be used when cellulite is present.

In some cases, mesotherapy is used to stimulate hair growth, but only for certain kinds of hair loss problems. Its primary cosmetic use is for reducing fat where it cannot be eliminated by diet and exercise.

Lipodissolve procedure is similar to mesotherapy but the injection is given deep into the corporeal fat layer and uses a larger needle. In both mesotherapy and lipodissolve, fat cells are drained rather than removed as they are with liposuction. Since these 2 procedures are so similar in function and result, the words mesotherapy and lipodissolve are often used interchangeably. These nonsurgical procedures have no downtime, unlike the surgical liposuction process.

How They Work

With mesotherapy, microinjections using very fine needles about the thickness of an eyelash target a customized "cocktail" of vitamins, amino acids, and medications into your problem areas just millimeters beneath the skin's surface layer. The primary component of this solution is the same as that found in soy lecithin. Lecithin allows your own body to release the fat within where it is burned as fuel. It is so effective that, in a specialized form, it is even used to increase circulation and reduce inflammation present in some serious medical conditions.

The procedure usually takes three or more treatments done within a few weeks of each other, and the results can be dramatic. Mesotherapy actually melts away the fat beneath the skin and shrinks the fat cells. When combined with a healthy combination of diet and exercise, this can be a solution for your fat loss, contouring, and cellulite problems.

Questions, Questions, Questions

Here are some of the most commonly asked questions about the procedure. If you have others, it is always best to discuss them with your doctor.

1. How quickly will I see results?

Some patients see results after the first treatment while others see results after several treatments. Mesotherapy and lipodissolve results for the body are measured in loss of inches rather than pounds. Remember, they are used mainly for body shaping rather than overall weight loss.

2. How many treatments will I need?

Everyone is different. Your treatment program will be customized for you based on your cellulite and fat deposits, and where they are located. Your doctor will be the best judge of how many treatments you need for maximum results.

3. How long will my results last?

Again, everyone is different. Many patients have found that, when used in combination with a healthy diet and exercise, the results can last a lifetime.

4. Is it painful?

Mesotherapy involves the use of a very thin needle that is about the thickness of an eyelash, so treatments are relatively pain free. Get assurances from your doctor that everything is done to ensure your comfort, including the application of an anesthetic cream, if necessary, to minimize any discomfort that you may feel.

5. Are there any side effects?

Side effects are minimal and generally disappear quickly. They are usually limited to redness, bruising, and swelling. Since mesotherapy and lipodissolve are delivered directly to specifically targeted areas, the possibility of drug interactions is significantly reduced. In some cases, the doctor will suggest that you not exercise or take any anti-inflammatory medications within the first twenty-four to forty-eight hours after a treatment.

6. When can I return to my normal activity?

Immediately. Since this is a nonsurgical procedure, there is no downtime and no special care required after treatment.

7. Are mesotherapy and lipodissolve safe?

Yes. These procedures have been used successfully for more than a half-century on tens of thousands of patients worldwide, and when used in their correct forms, have an excellent safety record.

8. How do I select the right person to do my meso-therapy and/or lipodissolve?

As with all cosmetic treatments, always make sure that the person performing any of these procedures is qualified to do them and ask how many times they have performed your specific treatment. Ask about certification and specific training in mesotherapy. If the doctor is not certified or experienced in these procedures, find someone who can meet these criteria. See Chapter 16 for more information about choosing your doctor.

9. Can anyone have mesotherapy and/or lipodisoolve?

Due to the mixture of vitamins, amino acids, and medications used, some patients cannot have this treatment. You cannot have mesotherapy and/or lipodissolve if you are pregnant, are an insulin-dependent diabetic, have a history of certain bleeding disorders, or take certain medications for heart disease. Discuss your medical/health history frankly and in depth with your doctor to decide if you can have this procedure.

10. How much does mesotherapy/lipodissolve cost?

This is a highly personalized procedure. The cost varies depending on which areas are treated and how extensive the problem is. You and your doctor will determine the best treatment plan for you and determine the number of treatments needed to get the most successful results.

Mesotherapy and Lipodissolve Results

The same patients mentioned earlier have the following to say after their mesotherapy and lipodissolve procedures.

"After mesotherapy, I lost eight inches and eleven pounds and the ten-minute treatments were easy."

Diane G., age 49, Real Estate Agent

"I am thrilled with the results. The nonsurgical treatments allowed me to continue my daily activities. After four treatments, I feel healthier and more confident since I have reduced the size and shape of my lower body."

Jennifer B., age 35, Retail Manager

"I was amazed at how the bulges disappeared after mesotherapy treatments."

Marie C., age 48, Receptionist

"My jaw line and the area under my chin look much more like they did decades ago. With the contouring, I look more youthful than I could have imagined."

Linda R., age 60, PR Consultant

Section Three

Summing It All Up

CHAPTER 16

Choosing a Doctor:
Your Most Important Decision

The doctor you choose to perform your skin rejuvenation and repair procedures is among the most important medical professionals that you will ever select. This is the person who will be selecting and performing the treatments that can change your appearance, who will affect others' perceptions of you, and who will participate in creating the personal image that you want for yourself.

A number of factors will help you to make a fully educated decision as to who that doctor should be:

- Your doctor should be highly skilled and knowledgeable about the procedures, treatments that will be done, and products that will be used, and should be well versed in the latest technology that is available.

- She should be an authority in her area and be a teaching professional who is asked to train other doctors about these procedures and treatments.

- This doctor should have performed a large number of procedures and treatments similar to the ones that you are seeking. It is always best when someone else is the guinea pig for a procedure. Don't be afraid to ask about others' results.

- A doctor's credentials are an excellent indication of his capabilities. These are proof of his trustworthiness and abilities, as assessed by his professional peers, and should be considered when making any medical decision.

Your Doctor's Qualifications

It is critical to understand your doctor's qualifications. Great cosmetic doctors are the product of many things. Among them is the general medical training that they have received, but this is just the beginning. Today's wide range of options for rejuvenation and other procedures requires a willingness to gain continuous education; to research your specific problems, if needed; and to become intuitive about which alternatives are the appropriate ones for you. These are in addition to a perfectionist's approach to the final results.

While general medical training is a fine basis for this, it is important to understand that most of your doctor's qualifications and capabilities in this field are the result of a respect for science and a desire to be the best possible cosmetic doctor.

This is a lifelong process. Since the progress in this field is so dynamic, your doctor will need to be flexible in adapting to newer, better procedures and products; open to adopting the ones that he has confidence in; and able to communicate effectively. Knowledge and expertise are relatively without value if your doctor cannot share information with you.

Ask your doctor if he or she gives seminars or trains others in the procedure that you are considering. Ask where your doctor learned the procedure and how long ago. If he is hesitant to tell you, find another doctor.

Cheapest Is Not Always Best

There is an old saying that goes, "The bitterness of low quality lasts longer than the sweetness of low price." Truer words were never spoken. This is your face and your body. Do you really want to make your decision based on who is less expensive?

Price should never be the primary consideration when you are weighing alternatives. It is far more important to evaluate the quality of the doctor, her experience, and credentials, and make a decision accordingly. This is not the place for bargain shopping.

Professional Atmosphere

The manner in which you are treated before you make your decision is a reflection of how you will be treated when you have procedures and require follow-up. The staff and the environment of the medical office are determined by the doctor. If you are not treated well when you are researching your treatments, you can probably be sure that nothing will change later. The doctor's attitudes and style are factors in all aspects of his or her office.

The standards that a doctor sets for his staff are the standards that will define your entire relationship.

Ask yourself the following questions:
- When you call, are you greeted professionally by the office staff?
- Are you made to feel that your call has value?
- Do your questions get answered promptly and satisfactorily?
- Are your requests for written information or brochures handled effectively?

- Are you satisfied with their handling of appointments and scheduling?

These are not trivial matters. They are an indication of how your relationship will proceed, and that the practice is operated professionally.

References and Testimonials

Talk to people who have had procedures done, and listen to what they have to say. It is important to remember that everyone's individual experience with a procedure, treatment, or product is just that. When you have something done, everything that you bring into the experience is specific to you.

At the same time, your doctor should be able to provide you with case histories or contact information so that you can talk to people who have had comparable procedures. Rejuvenation and repair are highly personal issues, but most people who are pleased with their results are willing to share their perspective.

Be Highly Sensitive to How the Doctor Answers Questions

The way to learn about a doctor is to ask many questions and listen carefully to the answers. Be open and proactive in asking about those things that you want and need to know. If you are not comfortable with how the doctor responds, reconsider your choice. No skilled doctor should be defensive about his responses; the best medical professionals are forthcoming and enthusiastic about answering. After all, this is the field that they have chosen, and if they are not willing to share their expertise with you, something is wrong.

At the very least, ask these questions:

1. Are you board certified?

This question should be the first one you ask. Plastic surgeons, dermatologists, and cosmetic surgeons must pass rigorous written and oral examinations to receive board certification.

2. How long have you being doing this procedure?

This will tell you if the doctor is the product of a series of weekend courses or is committed to keeping up with scientific advancement. Science and technology are always progressing. This means keeping up with new techniques and ongoing training are necessary to maintaining skills.

3. How many procedures (or patients) do you see in a year?

A popular doctor is probably a very capable doctor since most of his practice in this field comes from word of mouth.

4. Where did you train?

Great doctors often get their training from other great doctors. By doing this they can learn the principles, watch best practices from the masters, and make the procedure their own. Knowing where and with whom your doctor trained is valuable information.

5. Where do you perform your procedures?

Look for a doctor with a well-equipped treatment facility. Ask about equipment and how it is maintained.

6. How do you safeguard against complications?

Complications are rare when you select a highly qualified doctor, but it is important to know how your doctor deals with them on the rare occasions that they arise. Steer clear of any doctor who says, "My patients never have complications." Look for someone who acknowledges that complications do rarely occur since everyone is different. The response should be on the order of, "I take meticulous effort to avoid any complications. This takes extraordinary focus on the details. That is the way I operate my practice."

7. What are your follow-up procedures?

Procedures are not complete until the patient has a satisfactory follow-up experience. Look for a doctor who says that she (or someone from her staff) will call you within a day of having a treatment done, and who encourages you to call the office if you have any questions about your recovery. There should be a policy of immediate access for any problems or concerns. This is part of the doctor-patient relationship and is extremely important in your choice of a medical professional.

8. What is the price?

You should know the cost of your procedures and treatments before you are required to make a commitment. While this is no place for bargain shopping, you should be comfortable with the costs that you are incurring for both the initial treatment and for any maintenance that is required to meet your expectations. You need to be confident that once an understanding is reached, it will be honored and that the doctor will not cut corners.

When you have the answers that you are looking for, make your judgment based on credentials, skill level, and chemistry. That's right: if you do not feel that you and the doctor can work well together, move on. There are fine doctors about whom you are confident and comfortable. That is the foundation of a relationship that can help you to look your best.

CHAPTER 17

Face Value:

Deciding the Right Time for a Medical Intervention

By now, you have explored the alternatives and options that are described in this book and have seen yourself in the descriptions of the problems and case histories. You are an educated consumer regarding rejuvenation procedures and treatments that can turn back the clock to a time when you had smooth, clear skin without wrinkles and lines, red or brown spots, and—perhaps—before acne or rosacea caused you embarrassment or discomfort about your self-image.

You are probably asking yourself if you are ready to take the plunge and get your specific problems solved. If you are asking yourself whether you can afford it, you need to also ask yourself whether you can afford NOT to seek a better you.

Ask yourself these questions:

- Am I happy with my appearance?
- Does my face or body make me look older than I feel?
- Have sun damage or the results of other bad habits like smoking left their mark?
- Do the lines and wrinkles on my face show the stress of a lifetime?

- Am I a victim of acne and its aftermath, and am I ready to reverse its effects?
- Are rosacea or facial blood vessels causing me discomfort when I look in the mirror?
- Does unwanted hair make me uncomfortable?
- Do I want the look of a natural face-lift without the surgery?
- Are there areas of fat deposits that I can't seem to get rid of with diet and exercise?
- Is the texture and tone of my skin what it was when I was younger?
- Are the contours of my face appearing to give in to gravity by sagging or sinking?
- Do I want to get on the right path for a lifetime of great skin?

If the answer to any of these questions is "yes," then one or more of today's state-of-the-art procedures, treatments, and products are for you.

Now, ask yourself if you are looking for a solution that is safe, noninvasive, relatively pain free, and without downtime. That will help you to exclude anything that is surgical.

The next question is, "Do I want the freedom to change my mind and reverse the effects of my treatment, or do I want to do something permanent that cannot be changed without surgery?" That, too, can help you to exclude surgical alternatives.

Another test is to ask yourself if you want to be more competitive in the business environment, more comfortable in a social environment, and more satisfied every time you look in the mirror. If you answered "yes," you are an ideal candidate for treatment.

If you are weighing the cost of any procedure or treatment, it is critical to balance that with your answers. If you believe that looking more youthful, vibrant, healthy, and self-assured will make your life better, it is time for a consultation with your doctor to establish a treatment plan and start on the road to meeting your specific needs.

There will never be a better time than now. None of the problems and situations that you have defined will ever get any better without the right medical intervention.

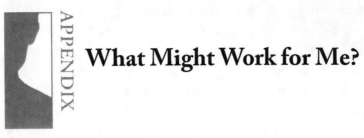

What Might Work for Me?

As you now know, cosmetic problems can be helped with many different treatments. To help you research possible treatment options for your particular needs I have listed on the following pages some of the most common cosmetic problems and their possible nonsurgical treatment options.

Problem	Possible Cosmetic Solution
Acne and acne scarring	• Chemical peels • Fraxel re:pair • Fraxel re:store • Injectable fillers • Laser treatments • Medications • Microdermabrasion
Baggy eyelids	• Fraxel re:pair • Fraxel re:store • Laser treatments • Thermage
Body contouring	• Mesotherapy/LipoDissolve • Smartlipo • Thermage
Broken blood vessels	• GentleWaves • IPL (intense pulsed light) • Laser treatments
Brown spots	• Chemical peels • Fraxel re:pair • Fraxel re:store • GentleWaves • IPL • Laser treatments
Cellulite	• Mesotherapy/LipoDissolve • Thermage
Crow's-feet	• Botox • Chemical peels • Fraxel re:pair • Fraxel re:store • Injectable fillers • Laser wrinkle reduction • Microdermabrasion • Thermage

Double chin or jowls	• Fraxel re:pair • Injectable fillers • Mesotherapy/LipoDissolve • Smartlipo • Thermage
Elongated ear lobes	• Injectable fillers
Excess or unwanted hair	• Electrolysis • IPL hair removal • Laser hair removal
Excessive sweating	• Botox
Facial Contouring	• Fraxel re:pair • Injectable fillers • Mesotherapy • Smartlipo • Thermage • VolumaLift
Facial veins	• GentleWaves • IPL • Laser treatments
Flabby or crepe-like skin	• Anti-aging skin care programs • Chemical peels • Fraxel re:pair • Fraxel re:store • Laser treatments • Microdermabrasion • Smartlipo
Forehead lines	• Botox • Fraxel re:pair • Fraxel re:store • Injectable fillers • Thermage

Frown lines	• Botox • Fraxel re:pair • Fraxel re:store • Injectable fillers • Laser treatments • Thermage
Hollow, sunken cheeks	• Injectable fillers • VolumaLift
Love handles	• Mesotherapy • Smartlipo • Thermage
Marionette or puppet lines	• Botox • Injectable fillers • Thermage
Melasma	• Fraxel re:store
Nasolabial lines	• Injectable fillers
Rosacea, redness, red spots	• GentleWaves • IPL • Laser treatments
Sagging neck	• Fraxel re:pair • Mesotherapy • Smartlipo • Thermage
Sallow skin	• Anti-aging skin care programs • Chemical peels • Fraxel re:pair • Fraxel re:store • GentleWaves • Laser treatments • Microdermabrasion • Thermage

Scars	• Chemical peels • Fraxel re:pair • Fraxel re:store • Injectable fillers • Laser treatments • Microdermabrasion
Turkey neck	• Mesotherapy • Smartlipo • Thermage
Under-eye circles	• Bleaching agents • Chemical peels • Fraxel re:pair • Fraxel re:store • Laser treatments • Thermage
Under-eye hollows	• Chemical peels • Injectable fillers • VolumaLift
Vertical lip lines	• Fraxel re:pair • Fraxel re:store • Injectable fillers

Informational Sources

While the entirety of this book is the work of Dr. Alexander J. Covey, the following publications and Web sites were instrumental sources to its development.

Books

Brandt, Fredric, MD with Patricia Reynoso. *Age-Less*. New York: HarperCollins, 2002.

Fairfield, James C., MD. *Erase the Years*. Terantum: Word Association Publishers, 2006.

Goldberg, David J., MD and Eva M. Herriott, PhD. *Light Years Younger*. Herndon: Capital Books Inc., 2003.

Irwin, Brandith, MD and Mark McPherson, PhD. *Your Best Face Without Surgery*. Carlsbad: Hay House, 2002.

Narins, Rhoda S., MD and Paul Jarrod Frank, MD. *Turn Back the Clock Without Losing Time*. New York: Three Rivers Press, 2002.

Web Sites

Botox.com
Restylane.com
Smartlipo.com
Volumalift.com

For more information on any of the subjects covered in this book, log on to

Eastendlasercare.com
Mesotherapynewyork.com
Volumaliftnewyork.com

Or contact the office of Dr. Alexander J. Covey to arrange for an appointment.

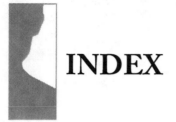

INDEX

chest. *See* brown spots; hair removal; redness, red spots

chin, double, 46, 120

chin, redness of, 71

chin, unwanted hair, 78

coenzyme Q10, 12

collagen

    bovine, 36–37

    deterioration of, 36–38, 41

    injections of, 41

    repair of, 12, 58–61

    replacement of, 40–41

    stimulating production of, 74, 76, 84–85, 87, 89–90, 95–96

CosmoDerm, 40–41

CosmoPlast, 40–41

crow's feet, 29, 63, 119

cystic acne. *See* acne

D

dark spots. *See* brown spots; redness, red spots

dermabrasion, 67, 83–88

dermal fillers. *See also* VolumaLift

    candidates for, 37–38

    current types of, 38–41

    downtime, 39, 42

    history of, 36–37

    ingredients of, 38–39

    results of, 39

    for treatment of acne, 39, 67

dermal layer. *See* skin

diet, 11–13

doctor, selection of

    credentials of, 108–109, 112

    prices of, 110, 113

microdermabrasion; Smartlipo MPX™; Thermage
forehead lines. *See also* laser treatments
    Botox, 27, 28, 29
    dermal fillers, 37, 40
    Thermage, 60, 71
fotofacial. *See* intense pulsed light (IPL)
fractioned laser resurfacing, 68–69. *See also* Fraxel re:pair;
    Fraxel re:store
Fraxel re:pair, 68–69, 95–97
Fraxel re:store, 75–76, 94–95, 96–97
freckles, 24, 74, 87. *See also* brown spots
frown lines. *See* lips

G
GentleWaves LED Photomodulation
    length of treatments, 88
    procedure, 87
    side effects, 88
glycolic acid. *See* chemical peels

H
hair growth
    causes of, 78
    stimulation of, 101
hair loss, 101
hair removal
    creams, 79
    electrolysis, 79
    generally, 77–79, 120
    intense pulsed light, 73
    shaving, 79
    waxing, 79
hair removal with laser
    frequency of treatment, 81

results of, 102, 103, 104–105
    safety of, 103
    side effects of, 103
    used for hair growth, 101
microdermabrasion
    amount of treatment, 87
    procedure, 67–68, 86
    for treatment of acne, 67, 87
migraine headaches, 26, 29
moisturizers, 84

N

nasolabial folds or lines, 39, 41, 46, 121. *See also* fillers,
        injectable
neck. *See also* laser treatments; mesotherapy; Smartlipo
        MPX™; Thermage
    bands, 29
    sagging, 121
    turkey, 57, 122
non-ablative laser treatments, 68. *See also* fractioned laser
        resurfacing

O

oil glands, enlarged, 74

P

paraffin, 36
peels. *See* chemical peels
Perlane, 38
photo-facials. *See* intense pulsed light (IPL)
photo rejuvenation. *See* intense pulsed light (IPL)
photothermolysis laser treatments, 67
physicians. *See* doctor, selection of

pigmented lesions. *See* brown spots; redness, red spots

pimples. *See* acne

polycystic ovary syndrome, 78

pores, size reduction of, 74

ptosis, 33–34

pulsed dye laser treatment

   deep wrinkles, 92

   length of treatment, 91

   maintenance, 91–92

   preparation for, 92

   procedure, 89–90

pulsed light. *See* intense pulsed light (IPL)

R

Radiesse, 40. *See also* dermal fillers

radiofrequency (RF) technology, 59

red lesions. *See* redness, red spots

redness, red spots

   causes of, 70–73, 76, 89, 96

   treatment of (*See* chemical peels; intense pulsed light
      (IPL))

Restylane, 38–39, 45, 46. *See also* dermal fillers

resurfacing, 68–69. *See also* laser treatments

Retin-A, 66

rhinophyma, 71. *See also* rosacea

rosacea

   description of, 71

   intense pulsed light (IPL) treatment, 73–74

   minimizing, 71–72

   pulsed dye laser treatment, 89

   treatment of, 72–73, 74–76, 121

cost of, 62
doctor selection, 62
downtime, 62
length of, 61
procedure, 58–59, 60–61
results of, 61, 62–63
safety of, 60
thighs
cellulite (*See* mesotherapy; Thermage)
fat (*See* Smartlipo MPX™)
skin tightening (*See* Thermage)
thin lips. *See* lips
turkey neck. *See* neck

U
underarms. *See* hair removal; sweating, excessive
unwanted hair. *See* hair removal

V
veins, facial. *See* spider veins
vertical lip lines. *See* lips
vitamins, 11, 12, 31, 42, 67, 101, 104
VolumaLift
alternatives, 48
cost of, 49
doctor selection, 48–49
downtime, 48
facial fat, 44, 46
how it works, 45–46
length of results, 47
length of treatment, 47
procedure, 45–46
results of, 47, 49
safety of, 46

W

waistline fat. *See* mesotherapy; Smartlipo MPX™
water, 9, 12–13, 18
whiteheads, 65
wrinkles, causes of, 16–17, 19
wrinkles, treatment of. *See* Botox; dermal fillers; laser
     treatments

Z

Zyderm, 36
Zyplast, 36

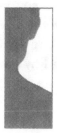

About the Author

Dr. Alexander Covey is a nationally renowned cosmetic surgeon, author, lecturer and the director of East End Laser Care in Manhattan, Southampton, and Center Moriches, New York. He is board certified in cosmetic surgery has been practicing medicine and performing cosmetic procedures since 1988. He is a diplomate of the American Board of Laser Surgery, the American Board of Internal Medicine, and a fellow of the American Academy of Cosmetic Surgery and the American Society for Laser Medicine and Surgery. He is also a member of the International Society of Cosmetic Laser Surgeons, the American College of Physicians, the American Medical Meso-Lipo Society, and the New York Medical Society. Dr. Covey is an attending physician at Peconic Bay Medical Center in Riverhead, New York.

Dr. Covey's long list of credentials and years of cumulative experience have earned him national recognition as an expert in the field of cosmetic surgery. He has dedicated himself to learning and teaching the latest and most advanced techniques in nonsurgical cosmetic treatments and gives informational seminars to physicians and patients about alternatives to surgical cosmetic procedures. Dr. Covey has been named one of the "Top Doctors in New York" for the last five years by the Castle Connolly Guide and has been named one of "America's Top Physician" by the Consumers' Research Council of America. He has written articles and has been quoted by numerous national and local publications.

Dr. Covey donates both resources and services to charities such as the Suffolk County Coalition Against Domestic Violence, for which he had been known to offer free treatments to domestic violence victims who couldn't otherwise afford them; Family Service League, which helps underprivileged children; and Ellen's Run to benefit breast cancer awareness and prevention. Dr. Covey lives in Long Island, New York, with his wife and children. In his free time he can sometimes be found incognito playing jazz piano at local restaurants and clubs.

CPSIA information can be obtained at www.ICGtesting.com
Printed in the USA
LVOW131546110213

319608LV00001B/70/P

9 781934 937969